Interpreting the
Electrocardiogram

Interpreting the Electrocardiogram

James S. Fleming
MD, FRCP

Consultant Cardiologist, Northern General, Hallamshire,
and Children's Hospitals, Sheffield, UK

1979
UPDATE BOOKS
LONDON · FORT LEE

Available in the United Kingdom and Eire from

Update Books Ltd
33/34 Alfred Place
London WC1E 7DP
England

Available outside the United Kingdom from

Update Publishing International Inc.
2337 Lemoine Avenue
Fort Lee, New Jersey 07024
USA

First Published 1979

© **Update Books Ltd, 1979**
© **James S. Fleming, 1979**

British Library Cataloguing in Publication Data

Fleming, James Samuel
    Interpreting the electrocardiogram.
    1. Electrocardiography
    I. Title
    616.1′2′0754   RC683.5.E5
 	
    ISBN 0–906141–05–2

ISBN 0 906141 05 2

Library of Congress Catalog
Card Number 78–74605

Printed in Great Britain by
Cox and Wyman Ltd, London, Fakenham and Reading

Contents

(The electrocardiograms for interpretation follow each chapter)

Preface

This book is intended primarily for the doctor who is confronted with an electrocardiogram and who wishes to make his own interpretation rather than to rely entirely upon the report of a specialist. The clinical use of the electrocardiogram is the sole concern here and no attempt is made to describe electrophysiology. It is hoped that by beginning with a description of the P wave and its abnormalities the reader will gain confidence and the desire to continue to subsequent sections as he realizes the simplicity of the approach. In a further attempt towards clarity and ease of reading, the text is liberally interspersed with line drawings, all originated by the author, and at the end of each section electrocardiograms are provided, illustrating the abnormalities which have been described.

Interest in the electrocardiogram has now spread from the cardiologist to a wide variety of hospital staff, including medical students, house officers, intensive care and coronary care nurses, and anaesthetists. Many general practitioners now record their own electrocardiograms and most have outpatient access to the electrocardiography department of their local hospitals. This book will provide a useful basis for their reading of the electrocardiogram and I hope convince them that its interpretation is well within their capabilities.

James Fleming
November 1978

1. Introduction

This book is concerned with the use of the electrocardiogram in clinical medicine. Before we begin, a word of warning! The electrocardiogram like any other diagnostic test must be taken together with all other information and not looked at in isolation. A patient with heart disease may have a normal electrocardiogram. Probably of greater importance is the normal patient who has an unusual electrocardiogram. The doctor inexperienced in the interpretation of the electrocardiogram does not realize the wide range of electrocardiograms which may be normal. A diagnosis should rarely, if ever, be made solely on the strength of 'abnormal electrocardiogram'.

The technical standard of recording the electrocardiogram must be high. Many mistakes will be made if a poor electrocardiograph is used. Even a good electrocardiograph with a high frequency response will give erroneous tracings if the stylus is wrongly adjusted. Correct positioning of the electrodes across the chest is, of course, essential and ST segment abnormalities cannot be assessed if the base line is wandering.

Because the electrocardiogram cannot be considered in isolation the best person to assess it is the physician looking after the case. He has all the contributory information available to him and should make best use of the electrocardiogram.

This book is designed to help the doctor understand better the meaning of a tracing so that the electrocardiogram becomes a more valuable clinical tool to him in caring for his patient. Perhaps the book will provide him with a companion to his study of this difficult subject.

Basic Principles

On the normal electrocardiogram, three deflections can be recognized during each cardiac cycle.

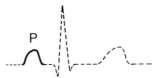

The P wave is caused by the depolarization wave spreading over both atria.

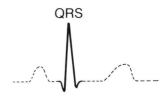

When the depolarization wave reaches the ventricles the QRS complex is written.

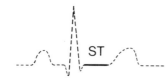

A period of electrical inactivity follows during which the electrocardiogram records the ST segment.

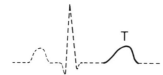

Finally, the ventricular muscle slowly recharges in preparation for the next heart beat and this repolarization of the ventricles appears as the T wave.

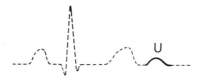

Occasionally, a small upright wave follows the T wave and this wave is called the U wave. The precise electrical events in the heart which cause the U wave are not known.

The standard electrocardiogram consists of 12 leads and before proceeding to the study of the normal and abnormal P wave the method of recording these leads should be understood.

Three bipolar leads are recorded (see Figure 1.1), leads I, II and III.

Three unipolar leads are also used: aVr, aVl and aVf. The unipolar lead picks up the potential at one point only, thus:

aVr records the potential at the right arm.
aVl records the potential at the left arm.
aVf records the potential at the left leg.

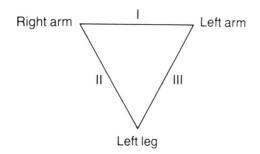

Figure 1.1. *Lead I: right arm to left arm. Lead II: right arm to left leg. Lead III: left arm to left leg.*

Finally six unipolar precordial leads are recorded in th positions shown (Figure 1.2).

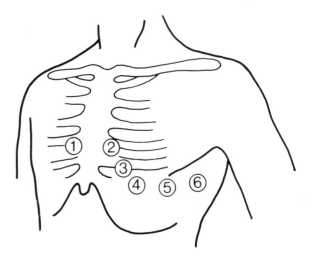

Figure 1.2. *Positions of precordial leads, V₁ to V₄.*

The tracings opposite (Figure 1.3) represent the normal 12-lead electrocardiogram.

The squared paper on which the electrocardiogram is recorded is also standard (Figure 1.4). The paper runs at a rate of 25 mm per second and the electrocardiograph is adjusted so that one millivolt of potential difference gives a vertical deflection of 10 mm.

Clinical interpretation of the electrocardiogram begins with the study of the P wave.

The impulse initiating each cardiac contraction arises in the sinoatrial (SA) node, close to the superior vena cava, and spreads outwards over the right and left atrium rather like a ripple in a pond when a stone has been thrown in.

The passage of the impulses over the atria writes the P wave on the electrocardiogram and the wave is usually best seen on standard lead II and precordial lead V₁.

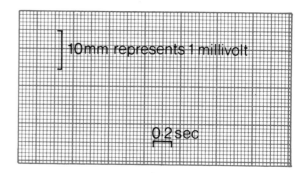

Figure 1.4. *Travelling horizontally, five large squares represent one second. One large square represents 0.2 seconds; one small square represents 0.04 seconds.*

2

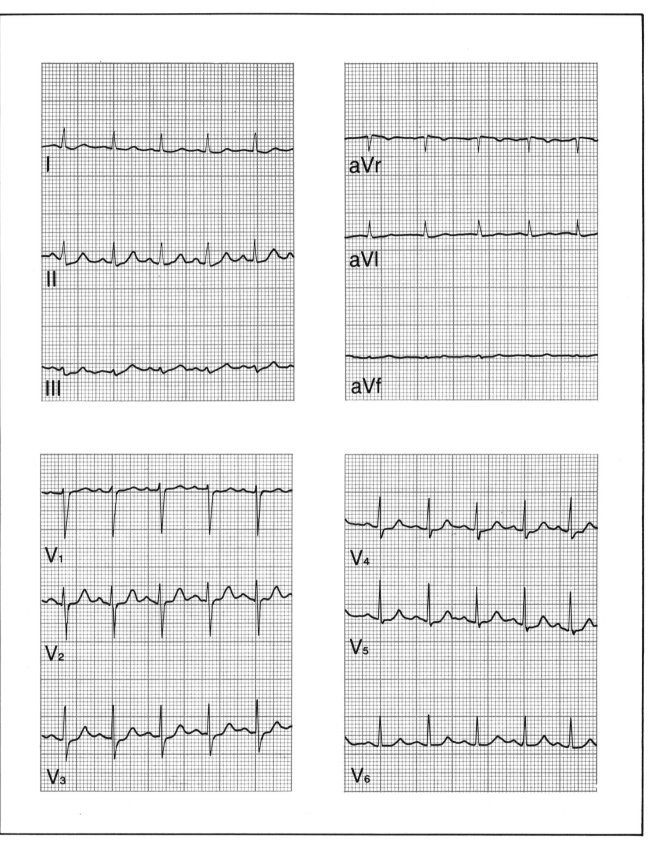

Figure 1.3. *The normal 12 lead electrocardiogram.*

2. The P wave

As already stated in Part 1, clinical interpretation of the electrocardiogram begins with the study of the P wave.

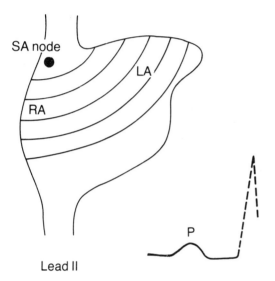

Figure 2.1. *Spread of excitation across atria from SA node. Normal P wave.*

The normal P wave (Figure 2.1) is upright in leads I and II, 0.08 seconds in duration (two small squares on the ECG paper) and not more than 2.5 mm in height.

In normal sinus rhythm every P wave is followed by a QRS complex and the regular sequence of P wave with closely following QRS complex provides electrocardiographic proof that the patient is in sinus rhythm.

Normal P wave in Lead I

The direction of passage of the impulse, from the SA node over the atria to the atrioventricular (AV) node, is downwards and to the left (Figure 2.2).

Movement to the left is always recorded as an upright deflection in lead I and the P wave is always upright in lead I under normal conditions.

Inverted P wave in Lead I

If the P wave appears inverted in lead I check that the right

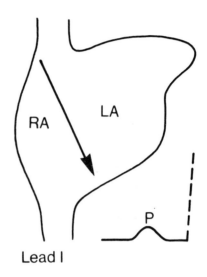

Figure 2.2. *Normal direction of spread of impulse from SA node over atria. P wave always upright in lead I.*

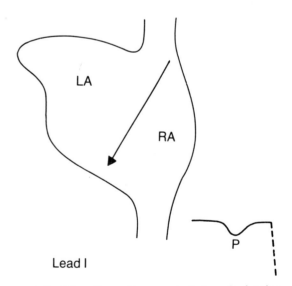

Figure 2.3. *Direction of spread of depolarization wave in mirror image dextrocardia. Inverted P wave in lead I.*

and left arm leads of the electrocardiograph have not been transposed. This is the most usual cause!

Assuming that the leads are correctly positioned, an inverted P wave in lead I means that the patient has mirror image dextrocardia.

In this condition the superior vena cava and right atrium are on the left side with the left atrium to the right, a mirror image of normal.

The wave of depolarization passes from the SA node downwards and to the right, resulting in an inverted P wave in lead I (Figure 2.3).

Right Atrial Hypertrophy (P pulmonale)

The hypertrophied myocardium of the right atrium has large movements of ions at a cellular level during the depolarization phase.

Right atrial hypertrophy is revealed on the electrocardiogram by a taller than normal P wave (Figure 2.4).

The duration of the wave is little affected by right atrial hypertrophy.

Causes of right atrial hypertrophy:

1. Disease of pulmonary vessels.
2. Tricuspid stenosis.
3. Tricuspid atresia.

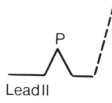

Lead II

Figure 2.4. *P pulmonale. P peaked, greater than 2.5 mm in height.*

Left Atrial Enlargement (P mitrale)

When there is enlargement of the left atrium the P wave is prolonged and bifid.

The first part of the P wave represents normal depolarization of the right atrium, the second peak on the P wave is produced by the depolarization wave spreading outwards over the enlarged left atrium (Figure 2.5).

A second clue to left atrial enlargement arises from the fact that the left atrium lies posteriorly, and its enlargement will therefore result in a large depolarization wave travelling posteriorly towards the end of atrial depolarization. This posteriorly directed wave is best seen in precordial lead V_1 (Figure 2.6).

If precordial lead V_1 shows a large negative deflection towards the end of the P wave, left atrial enlargement is present.

Causes of P mitrale include:

1. Left atrial enlargement.
2. Mitral valve disease.

3. Left ventricular failure.

4. Occasionally a notched P wave is caused by som fibrosis in the atria interrupting the smooth passage of th depolarization wave. A notched P wave under these ci cumstances does not indicate left atrial enlargement.

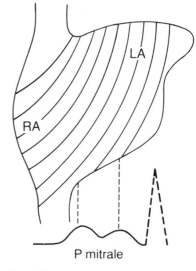

P mitrale

Lead II

Figure 2.5. *P mitrale. Enlarged left atrium produces second peak on P wave. P notched, over 0.12 seconds in duration (more than three small squares).*

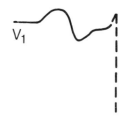

Figure 2.6. *Left atrial enlargement. Depolarization of left atrium produces a wave travelling away from V_1 lead position resulting in a large negative component to the P wave.*

Atrial Extrasystole

An atrial extrasystole occurs when some focus in the atria other than the SA node, initiates the atrial depolarization wave.

The depolarization wave will then travel over the atria in a different direction from that taken when the impulse arises in the SA node.

The P wave of an atrial extrasystole is of an unusual shape (Figure 2.7).

The significance of atrial extrasystole:

1. Often present in a normal heart.

2. Frequent bursts of atrial extrasystoles in a patient with mitral stenosis may indicate that atrial fibrillation will soon occur.

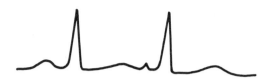

Figure 2.7. Atrial extrasystole. P wave of unusual shape preceding a normal QRS complex.

Nodal Rhythm

When the AV node takes over the pacemaker function of the heart from the SA node the wave of depolarization spreads upwards over the atria.

This change in direction results in a change in the direction of the P wave in leads II and III (Figure 2.8).

The inverted P wave may appear before, during or after the inscription of the QRS complex, depending upon the precise site of the origin of the impulse.

If the highest part of the AV node initiates the impulse, then the atria are depolarized slightly before the impulse of depolarization reaches the ventricles and the inverted P wave appears before the QRS complex.

A low nodal site of origin has the opposite effect, and the inverted P wave occurs after the QRS complex.

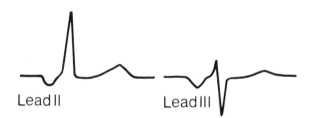

Figure 2.8. Nodal rhythm. P inverted in leads II and III. PR interval less than 0.12 seconds.

The PR Interval

This important interval gives an estimate of the state of the conducting system of the heart.

The PR interval is measured from the onset of the P wave to the onset of the QRS complex (Figure 2.9) and represents the time taken for the impulses from the SA node to pass down to and through the AV node to the bundle of His and to begin depolarization of the ventricles.

A PR interval greater than 0.22 seconds indicates first degree heart block.

Causes of first degree heart block include:

1. Acute myocarditis where a long PR interval is seen frequently during acute rheumatic fever.

2. Drug effects (digitalis, quinidine, potassium).

3. Degeneration of the conducting system.

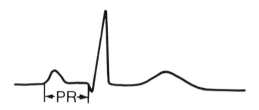

Figure 2.9. PR interval. PR normally not greater than 0.22 seconds (slightly more than five small squares).

Summary

Normal P wave:

1. Upright in leads I and II.

2. Duration of 0.08 seconds (two small squares).

3. Not more than 2.5 mm in height.

Inverted P wave in leads I and II (in a patient in sinus rhythm):

1. Right and left arm leads have been transposed.

2. Mirror image dextrocardia.

P pulmonale:

1. Tall triangular P wave more than 2.5 mm in height.

2. Right atrial hypertrophy.

P mitrale:

1. P wave notched and 0.12 seconds (three small squares) or more in duration.

2. Left atrial enlargement.

Atrial extrasystole:

P wave of abnormal shape appearing earlier than the next expected normal P wave, usually followed by a normal QRS complex.

Nodal rhythm:

1. P wave inverted in leads II and III.

2. PR interval less than 0.12 seconds (three small squares).

PR interval:

1. Measured from beginning of P to beginning of QRS complex.

2. Normally less than 0.22 seconds (not more than 5.5 small squares).

7

2. Electrocardiograms for Interpretation

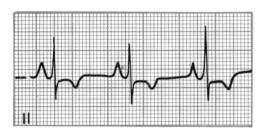

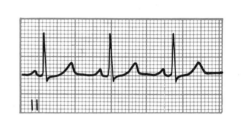

Normal P wave.

This patient has severe right ventricular hypertrophy.

This has caused right atrial hypertrophy and the electrocardiogram shows tall triangular P waves (P pulmonale).

Compare these with the normal P wave.

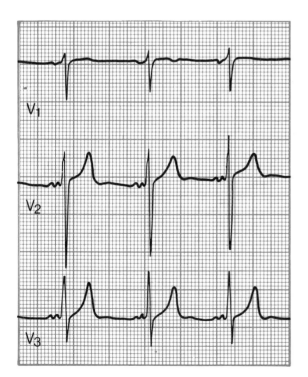

A good example of P mitrale in a female patient aged 30 who had severe mitral valve stenosis.

Note the negative terminal portion of the P wave in lead V_1 and the broad notched P wave in leads V_2 and V_3.

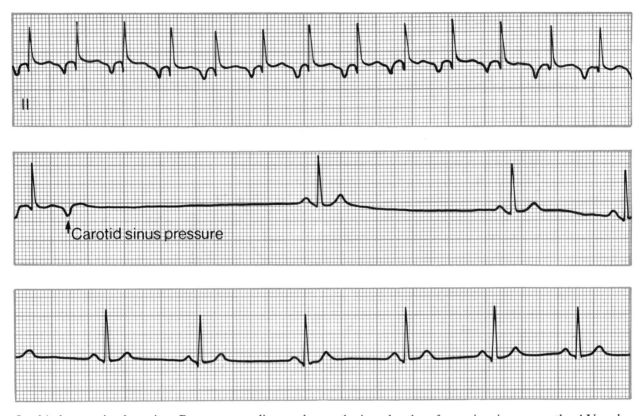

In this long strip there is a P wave preceding each QRS complex.

The lead recorded in this case is lead II showing an inverted P wave in the first 14 complexes.

An inverted P wave in lead II suggests that the impulse is spreading upwards over the atria and that the impulse therefore arises in or near the AV node. Carotid sinus pressure was applied which stimulated the vagus nerve and suppressed the nodal focus.

The second half of the tracing shows that carotid sinus pressure has terminated this nodal rhythm and sinus rhythm has been restored.

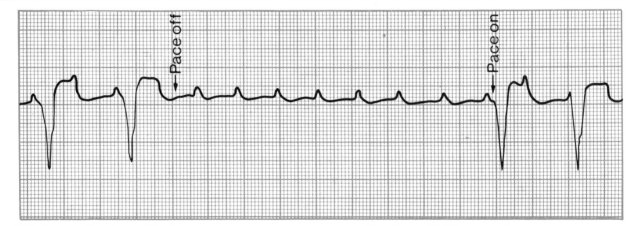

This is complete heart block.

The first two QRS complexes have been stimulated electrically by an artificial pacemaker. The pacemaker was then switched off for a brief period and regular P waves but no QRS complexes are seen. The artificial pacemaker was then switched on again and the last two complexes show the ventricles being paced by the artificial pacemaker.

The diagnosis is complete heart block in a case of acute myocardial infarction, requiring artificial pacemaking. In three days normal sinus rhythm returned in this patient and the artificial pacemaking electrode was later removed.

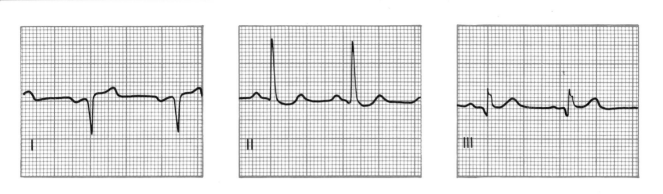

Standard leads I, II and III in a man aged 25. Each P wave is followed by a QRS complex and the PR interval is constant at 0.2 seconds. This is obviously sinus rhythm.

The P wave is inverted in Lead I and there had been no mistake in the attachment of the leads during the recording of the electrocardiogram, therefore indicating dextrocardia.

In mirror image dextrocardia the viscera in the abdomen are also in the mirror image of their usual position. In fact, this young man complained of severe pain in the left iliac fossa and an acutely inflamed appendix was removed from its position in the left lower abdomen. The stomach is of course on the right side and the liver on the left in this condition.

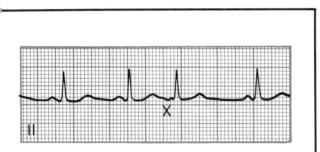

One atrial extrasystole (X).

Unusual shaped P wave followed by normal QRS.

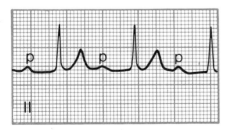

Prolonged PR interval.

PR measures 0.4 seconds (10 small squares. Upper limit of normal is 5.5 small squares).

This patient had acute rheumatic fever but there are other possible causes of a long PR interval, e.g. excess digitalis, quinidine, or degeneration of the conducting tissue.

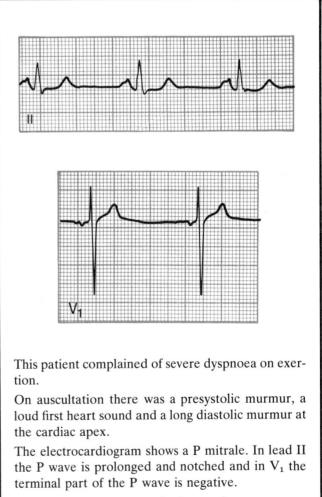

This patient complained of severe dyspnoea on exertion.

On auscultation there was a presystolic murmur, a loud first heart sound and a long diastolic murmur at the cardiac apex.

The electrocardiogram shows a P mitrale. In lead II the P wave is prolonged and notched and in V_1 the terminal part of the P wave is negative.

The diagnosis here was mitral stenosis.

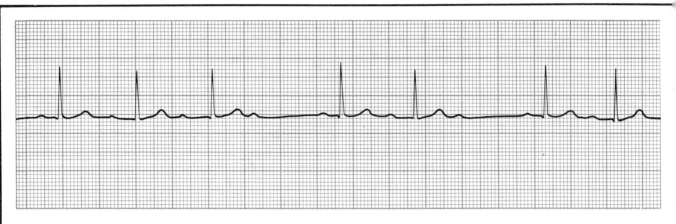

A more advanced degree of heart block.

The fourth P wave on the tracing is not conducted to the ventricles.

Note the progressive lengthening of the PR interval prior to the dropped beat. (This will be discussed in more detail in Part 10.)

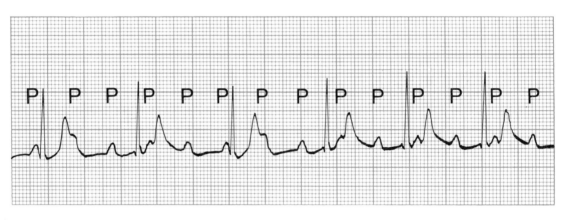

Normal P waves and normal QRS and T complexes.

The P waves are occurring at a faster rate than the QRS complexes and the PR interval is completely variable.

This is an example of complete heart block, the atrial impulses are not conducted to the ventricles.

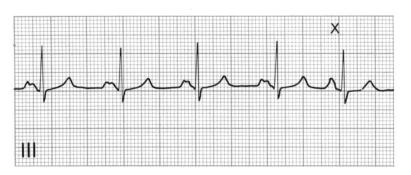

A good example of P mitrale.

The P waves are abnormally wide and notched. The last P wave has a different appearance and occurs early.

This last P wave is an atrial extrasystole.

3. The QRS Complex

The principal deflection of the electrocardiogram is the QRS complex (Figure 3.1), and alterations in the QRS waves provide information of great clinical value.

In healthy subjects the QRS complex is affected little, if at all, by emotion, hyperventilation, excitement and the host of other physiological changes which may so often affect the ST and T waves.

Abnormalities of the QRS complexes are of the greatest importance and usually indicate underlying disease, the nature of which may also be apparent from recognition of characteristic patterns.

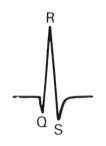

Figure 3.1.

The Normal QRS Complex

The QRS complex is inscribed as the wave of depolarization sweeps across the ventricles.

The impulse initiating each ventricular contraction spreads from the atrioventricular (AV) node into the bundle of His and is rapidly conducted down this bundle of specialized conduction tissue to the right and left bundle branches and thereafter to the Purkinje tissues of both ventricles. In this way, a wave of depolarization spreads into and through the myocardium of both ventricles and the passage of this wave through the ventricles produces the QRS deflections on the electrocardiogram.

In the normal heart the process of depolarization of the ventricles always begins at the interventricular septum on the left ventricular side and spreads from left to right as shown by arrow 1 (Figure 3.2).

Now consider what lead V_1 will record at the moment in time when the wave 1 (Figure 3.2) is present.

The position of lead V_1 on the patient's chest is such that this wave is travelling towards V_1.

An upward (positive) deflection is therefore recorded by

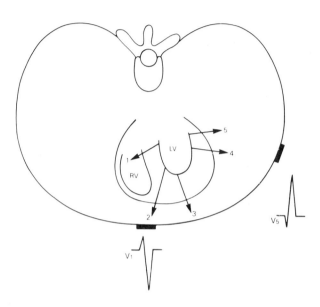

Figure 3.2. *Explanation of the shape of the QRS complex in leads V_1 and V_5.*

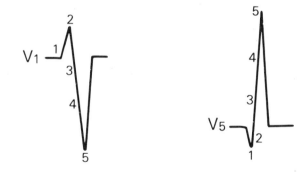

Figure 3.3. *Normal QRS in V_1 and V_5.*

the electrocardiograph when recording from the V_1 position. (1 in V_1, Figure 3.3).

The situation is different for lead V_5. Wave 1 (Figure 3.2) is travelling *away* from V_5, and lead V_5 will record a negative deflection at the moment in time that V_1 is recording a positive deflection.

Arrows 2, 3, 4 and 5 (Figure 3.2) indicate the direction of spread of the ventricular depolarization wave at later stages of the activation of the ventricles, and the deflection produced on the electrocardiogram at these stages is indicated for V_1 and V_5 (Figure 3.3).

An upward or positive deflection indicates that the depolarization wave is travelling towards the lead at that time, and a downward or negative deflection indicates that the wave is travelling away from that lead.

The Terminology of the QRS Complex

The use of capital letters or small letters has little significance. Small deflections are usually given small letters, but many authorities use capital letters regardless of size, for the purpose of simplicity (see Figures 3.4 and 3.5).

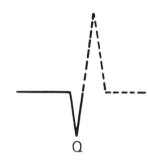

Figure 3.4. *Q wave: the initial downward deflection of the QRS complex.*

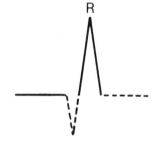

R wave: the first upward deflection.

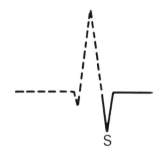

S wave: the initial negative deflection following the R wave.

Normal Values for the Adult

The normal QRS complex does not exceed 0.10 seconds duration (two and a half small squares) in any lead.

The R wave in V_5 and V_6 is less than 26 mm (less than 26 small squares) in height.

The sum of R wave in lead V_5 or V_6 and S wave in V_1 is les than 35 mm.

The R wave in the left leg lead, aVf, is less than 20 mm i height.

Many factors may influence the potential changes picke up at the body surface and recorded in the electro cardiogram. For example, obesity, hyperinflated lungs an pericardial effusion will all reduce the conductivity of th body and will tend to give a small QRS complex.

The normal values for the size of the QRS complex can b used only as a guide and the individual patient must b considered in the interpretation of each electrocardiogram e.g. is the patient obese, is there emphysema?

In childhood QRS waves may be large and the range o normality is considerable.

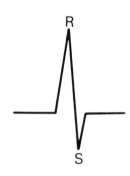

Figure 3.5. *In this tracing the initial deflection is upwards. The succeeding downward deflection is therefore an S wave and not a Q wave.*

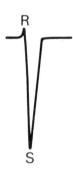

Similarly in this example the downward deflection is an S wave as there is a preceding R wave. If the initial deflection is upwards, no matter how small this R wave, then the succeeding downward deflection is an S wave.

The QRS Axis

The direction taken by the depolarization wave as it spreads across the ventricles is called the QRS axis.

The exact direction of the wave obviously changes from moment to moment during ventricular depolarization and therefore the QRS axis is the *average* direction taken throughout the whole process of ventricular depolarization.

The direction of the wave is usually determined as it

14

ppears when looking at the patient from in front (frontal plane view) (Figure 3.6).

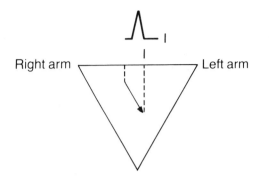

Figure 3.6. *If the wave of depolarization through the ventricles is in the direction shown by the arrow, standard lead I will record an upward, positive deflection. In lead I all waves travelling towards the left arm are recorded as positive.*

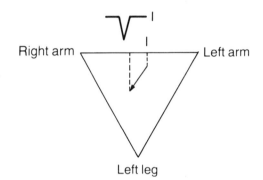

In this example lead I will record a negative deflection.

The normal QRS axis for adults lies within the limits -30 to $+90$ degrees (Figure 3.7).

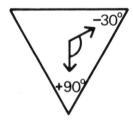

Figure 3.7 *Limits of normal QRS axis.*

Method for the Determination of the QRS Axis

The QRS axis may be determined from inspection of the standard leads using the reasoning explained above for each lead. However, a simpler procedure (Figures 3.8 and 3.9) exists:

1. Find the standard lead in which the area of the QRS above the isoelectric line is equal, or nearly equal, to the area below the isoelectric line. This indicates that the average direction of spread of the depolarization wave is at right angles to that lead. Draw a line on the diagram at right angles to that lead to represent the QRS axis.

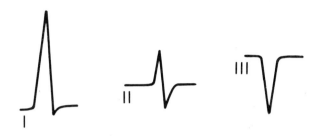

Figure 3.8. *This example should make the procedure clear. The areas above and below the isoelectric line are equal in II.*

A line is therefore drawn at right angles to II (Figure 3.9a).

2. Now look at the other standard leads. The QRS axis will point towards the lead where the main area of the QRS is above the isoelectric line. An arrow may now be drawn on the line in the diagram indicating the direction taken by the depolarization wave.

The main area of the QRS is above the isoelectric line in I. This means that the QRS axis produces a positive deflection in I, i.e. the depolarization wave is travelling towards the left arm.

An arrow can now be placed on the drawn line, indicating the direction of the QRS axis (Figure 3.9b).

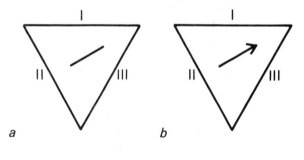

Figure 3.9.

Left Ventricular Hypertrophy

By far the largest mass of myocardium is contained in the walls of the left ventricle and the normal QRS complex is predominantly a result of left ventricular depolarization. In the presence of left ventricular hypertrophy, therefore, no striking change is to be expected in the shape of the QRS complexes. The hypertrophied muscle produces a larger than normal depolarization wave and this is recorded as a QRS complex of normal configuration but of increased magnitude.

With more severe left ventricular hypertrophy, repolarization of the ventricle is affected. Probably the pressure in the inner layers of the left ventricular myocardium becomes so high that during systole all coronary flow to this part is interrupted.

The ST and T waves of the electrocardiogram are recorded during ventricular repolarization and when repolarization is affected by left ventricular hypertrophy these waves become abnormal (Figures 3.10, 3.11 and 3.12).

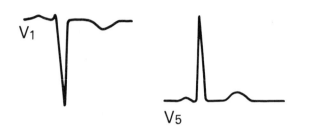

Figure 3.10. *Grade 1 changes of left ventricular hypertrophy. Voltage of QRS increased. Usually S wave is deep in V_1 and R is tall in V_5. Sum of S in V_1 and R in V_5 greater than 35 mm.*

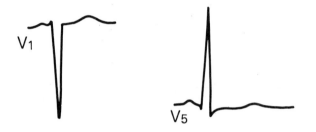

Figure 3.11. *Grade 2 left ventricular hypertrophy. Large voltage QRS, slight ST depression. T wave decreased in amplitude in V_5 and biphasic (initial part negative, later part positive).*

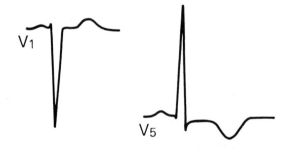

Figure 3.12. *Grade 3 left ventricular hypertrophy (severe). Large voltage QRS complexes. ST depression in V_5. Deep T inversion in V_5.*

Other Electrocardiographic Signs Occasionally Found in Left Ventricular Hypertrophy

Left Axis Deviation

A QRS axis further to the left than −30 degrees is, by definition, 'left axis deviation'.

When the electrocardiogram shows left axis deviation (Figure 3.13) the depolarization wave is taking a very abnormal pathway over the ventricles. The most usual cause is fibrosis of the ventricular muscle.

The finding of left axis deviation is by no means invariable in left ventricular hypertrophy and indeed, in children left axis deviation due to left ventricular hypertrophy is rare.

Left axis deviation, seen often in adults with severe left ventricular hypertrophy, implies considerable fibrosis of the left ventricular muscle in addition to the hypertrophy.

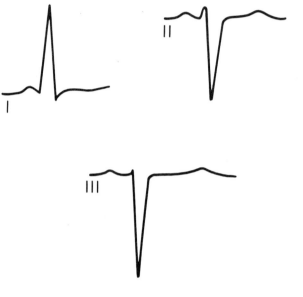

Figure 3.13.

Left Bundle Branch Block (Figure 3.14)

One cause of left bundle branch block is the interruption of the left bundle branch by a patch of fibrosis.

In severe left ventricular hypertrophy considerable fibrosis may follow, and in advanced left ventricular hypertrophy left bundle branch block may be seen on the electrocardiogram. Unfortunately, when the left bundle branch is blocked the appearance of the electrocardiogram is similar for all conditions causing the block.

It is difficult to make a confident electrocardiographic diagnosis of left ventricular hypertrophy and to exclude other pathologies such as myocardial infarction, cardiomyopathy, etc., when the pattern is that of left bundle branch block.

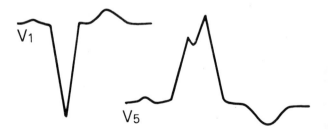

Figure 3.14.

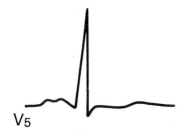

V_5

Figure 3.15.

P Mitrale (Figure 3.15)

A P mitrale may be seen in patients with left ventricular hypertrophy. It indicates an enlarged left atrium and is not specific for mitral valve disease.

Summary

Normal QRS:

1. Duration of 0.10 seconds or less (two and a half small squares).

2. Sum of R in V_5 or V_6 and S in V_1 less than 35 mm.

3. R in aVf less than 20 mm.

4. Small R in V_1 and small Q in V_5 is usual (septal depolarization).

5. Voltage variable within fairly wide limits.

QRS axis:

The direction taken by the ventricular depolarization wave. Normally lies within the range of -30 to $+90$ degrees.

Left ventricular hypertrophy:

Grade 1. Increased voltage of QRS.

Grade 2. Increased voltage of QRS with slight ST depression and biphasic T wave.

Grade 3. Increased voltage of QRS with ST depression and T wave inversion.

Other features which may, in appropriate patients, indicate left ventricular hypertrophy:

1. Left axis deviation.

2. Left bundle branch block.

3. P mitrale.

3. Electrocardiograms for Interpretation

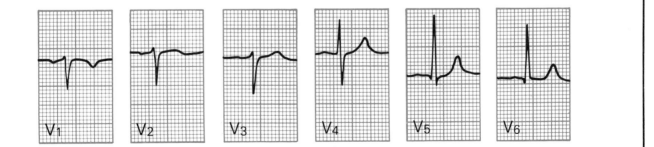

Normal QRS complexes in the precordial leads of a healthy adult.

Note the small R wave in V_1 becoming progressively taller as we move across the chest from V_1 to V_6.

V_5 and V_6 show the normal small Q waves in these leads produced by the septal depolarizing wave travelling from left to right.

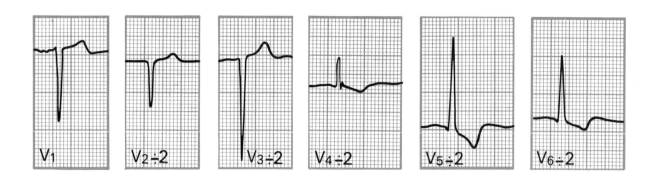

Severe left ventricular hypertrophy.

Note that precordial leads V_2, V_3, V_4, V_5 and V_6 are labelled as being recorded at half sensitivity. Thus the voltage of the R wave in V_5, for example, is not 23 mm but double this, i.e. 46 mm.

In addition to the ST and T segment changes indicating severe left ventricular hypertrophy there is the suggestion of a P mitrale, most obvious in lead V_1.

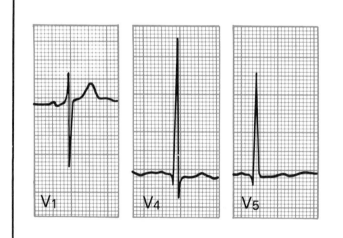

Grade 2 left ventricular hypertrophy.

Large QRS voltages ($SV_1 + RV_5 = 41$ mm). ST depression and biphasic T waves.

Grade 3 (severe) left ventricular hypertrophy.

Large QRS voltage. Depressed ST segment and inverted T wave.

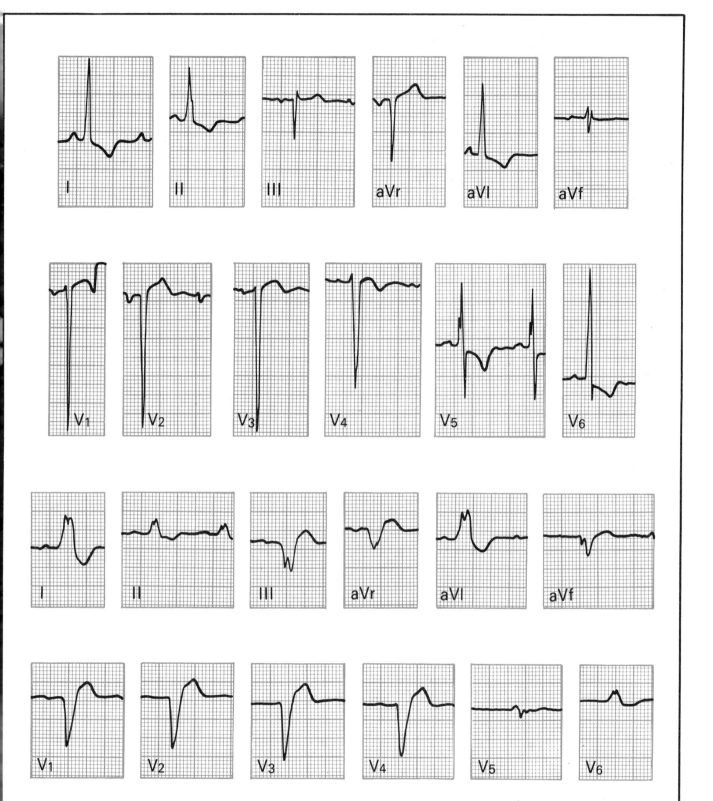

Two very interesting electrocardiograms, recorded from the same patient. There is an interval of one month between recordings.

In the first tracing all the electrocardiographic signs of severe left ventricular hypertrophy are present including large voltage QRS complexes, T wave inversion and ST segment abnormalities.

The second tracing shows left bundle branch block. If this second tracing alone had been available it would not have been possible to make the diagnosis of left ventricular hypertrophy from the electrocardiogram.

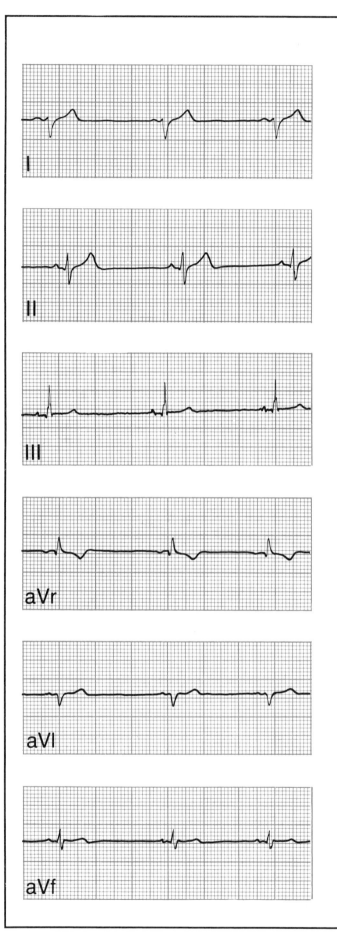

The QRS complex is dominantly negative in lead I and positive in lead III. This is right axis deviation: the QRS axis is +150 degrees.

Right axis deviation may indicate right ventricular hypertrophy, but this tracing was recorded from a seven-year-old boy and in youth right axis deviation is a frequent normal finding.

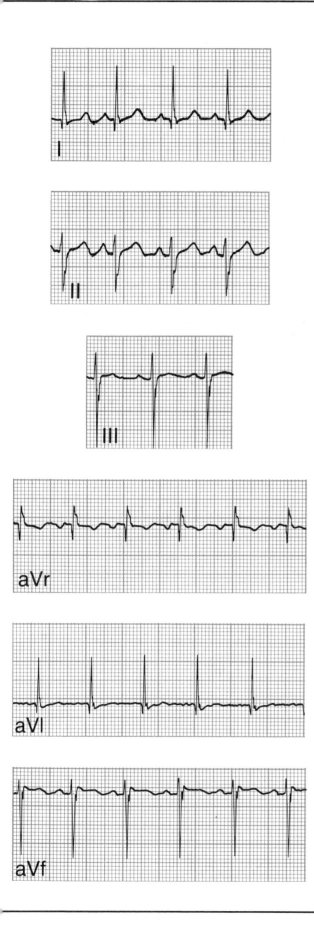

The QRS is dominantly negative in lead II and very negative in lead III. The mean QRS axis is −60 degrees.

This electrocardiogram was recorded from a six-year-old boy with an ostium primum atrial septal defect, but no left ventricular hypertrophy.

Left axis deviation does not always indicate hypertrophy.

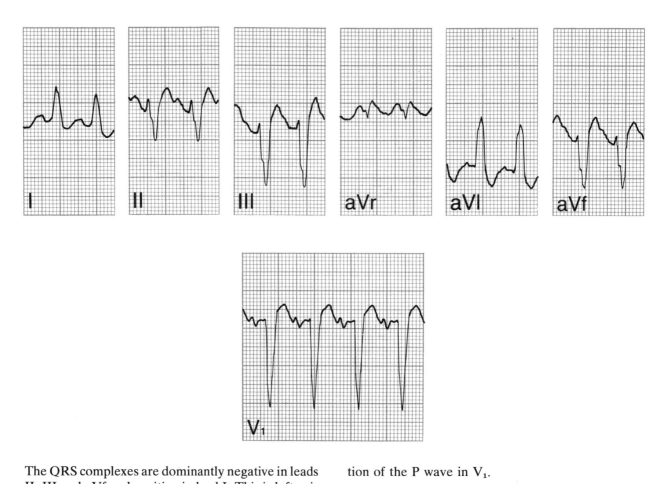

The QRS complexes are dominantly negative in leads II, III and aVf and positive in lead I. This is left axis deviation: the QRS axis is −60 degrees. The P wave is rather broad and there is a terminal negative deflection of the P wave in V_1.

This patient suffered from severe ischaemic heart disease with left ventricular failure and consequent enlargement of the left atrium.

4. Conditions Affecting the Right Side of the Heart

The wall of the right ventricle is much thinner than that of the left ventricle.

The QRS complex, which represents depolarization of both ventricles, is influenced mainly by the large bulk of myocardium of the left ventricle, the electrical forces of which swamp those arising from the right ventricle.

Right Ventricular Hypertrophy

Although the electrocardiogram is the most reliable clinical tool for the detection of right ventricular hypertrophy, for the reasons mentioned above minor degrees will not be detected.

Furthermore, in the presence of left ventricular hypertrophy, considerable degrees of right ventricular hypertrophy may be present without producing any characteristic electrocardiographic changes.

Changes in the Electrocardiogram Produced by Right Ventricular Hypertrophy

The presence of one or more of the following abnormalities in the electrocardiogram suggests the diagnosis of right ventricular enlargement.

Right Axis Deviation

Right axis deviation is an early sign of right ventricular hypertrophy.

The QRS complex represents the spread of the depolarization wave simultaneously over the left and right ventricles, and in the normal heart the direction of this wave is chiefly determined by the greater muscle mass of the left ventricle.

The effect of large electrical forces from a hypertrophied right ventricle is to swing the average direction of the depolarization wave in the direction of the hypertrophied chamber, i.e. to the right.

The QRS axis becomes recognizably abnormal only when the forces from the right ventricle are sufficiently large to cause the QRS axis to be greater than +90 degrees.

The arrow (see Figure 4.1), representing the average direction of spread of the ventricular depolarization wave, is in this case pointing downwards and to the right.

In lead I this arrow is seen as a current travelling towards

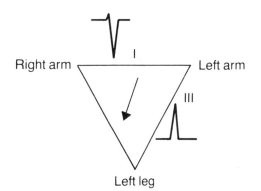

Figure 4.1. *Right axis deviation.*

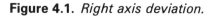

the right arm and the main area of the QRS complex in lead I is therefore negative.

Lead III records a large upright deflection since the direction of the wave is towards the left leg, and lead III records as positive all waves towards the leg.

The normal limits for the QRS axis lie between −30 and +90 degrees. Right ventricular hypertrophy must swing the axis to beyond +90 degrees before the axis becomes recognizably abnormal—unless, of course, in the individual patient a change in the axis can be detected from comparison with an electrocardiogram taken in the past.

Tall R waves in Leads V₁ and V₂

The right ventricle lies to the right and *in front of* the left ventricle (Figure 4.2).

During depolarization of the ventricles the forces from the hypertrophied right ventricle are large and, directed anteriorly, are travelling towards precordial leads V_1 and V_2.

The large electrical forces from the hypertrophied right ventricle are therefore recorded as large upright deflections in V_1 and V_2 (Figure 4.3).

T wave Inversions in V₁, V₂ and V₃

Inversion of the T waves in the anterior precordial leads represents a change in right ventricular repolarization and this usually accompanies severe right ventricular hypertrophy.

When tall R waves in V_1 and V_2 are accompanied by

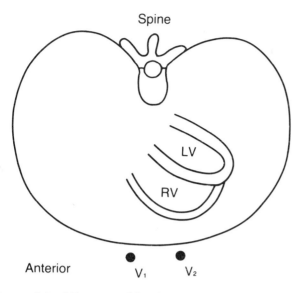

Posterior

Spine

LV

RV

Anterior V_1 V_2

Figure 4.2. *Diagram of horizontal section of body to illustrate the anterior position of the right ventricle.*

inverted T waves in these leads the electrocardiographic diagnosis is right ventricular hypertrophy and strain. (T wave changes will be considered more fully when ventricular repolarization is described in Part 8.)

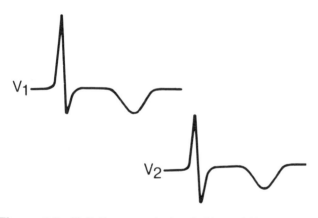

V_1

V_2

Figure 4.3. *Tall R waves in leads V_1 and V_2, indicating right ventricular hypertrophy. In general, when the ratio R/S in V_1 is greater than 1, right ventricular hypertrophy is present.*

Right Axis Deviation Accompanied by an RSR¹ Complex in V_1

When the right ventricle has enlarged as a result of pumping an increased volume of blood, as in atrial septal defect, the usual finding is an RSR¹ complex in V_1 (Figure 4.4). This is termed incomplete right bundle branch block by some authorities.

The shape of the QRS complexes in leads I and V_1 resembles that of right bundle branch block, but the duration of the entire QRS complex is less than 0.12 seconds (less than three small squares).

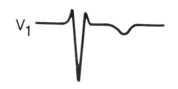

V_1

Figure 4.4. *RSR¹ complex in V_1. QRS duration less than 0.12 seconds (less than three small squares). Incomplete right bundle branch block.*

Bundle branch block is not present if the QRS complex duration is less than 0.12 seconds and this appearance cannot be called right bundle branch block for this reason.

Therefore, some authorities use the term incomplete right bundle branch block to describe the appearance of a terminal S wave in lead I with a terminal R¹ wave in lead V₁ when the QRS duration is less than 0.12 seconds.

The initial upward deflection is termed R, as usual.

The downward deflection following R is S. Again this is the routine terminology for the waves of the electrocardiogram. However, the S wave is followed by an upward deflection. This second upward deflection is called an R¹ wave.

It has been suggested that two types of right ventricular enlargement may be diagnosed from the electrocardiogram. Right ventricular hypertrophy due to a pressure overload, as in pulmonary valve stenosis, is characterized by tall R waves in V_1 and V_2, and right ventricular enlargement from a volume overload, as in atrial septal defect, is characterized by an RSR¹ complex in V_1.

Acute Right Ventricular Strain

Sudden onset of right ventricular strain occurs most characteristically with a large pulmonary embolus.

The electrocardiogram is often normal in this condition but when changes of right ventricular strain do appear the electrocardiogram gives valuable diagnostic aid.

One or more of the following abnormalities may occur:

1. Change in direction of the mean QRS axis to the right with gradual recovery to a more normal direction over the ensuing days.

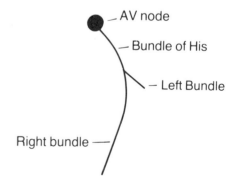

AV node

Bundle of His

Left Bundle

Right bundle

Figure 4.5.

2. Appearance of a small P pulmonale.

3. Inversion of T waves in precordial leads V_1, V_2, V_3 and V_4.

4. Appearance of an RSR^1 complex in V_1 and V_2.

5. Q waves may appear in III and aVf.

When electrocardiographic abnormalities do appear in pulmonary embolism the changes are usually maximal soon after the acute incident and the electrocardiogram may well revert to normal within a few days of the embolism.

Bundle Branch Block

The impulse initiating depolarization comes to the ventricles down the bundle of His and through the right and left branches (see Figure 4.5).

When conduction is interrupted in either of the bundle branches, bundle branch block is present and the depolarization wave takes an abnormally slow course through the myocardium of the region involved by the block.

As a result of the slow spread of the ventricular depolarization wave the electrocardiogram records a prolonged QRS complex.

A QRS complex of 0.12 seconds (three small squares) or more indicates bundle branch block.

Right Bundle Branch Block (Figure 4.6)

In right bundle branch block spread of the depolarization wave into the right ventricle is delayed.

Depolarization of the right ventricle now takes place after the left, and the terminal portion of the QRS complex is written by right ventricular depolarization alone.

The right ventricle lies to the right and in front of the left ventricle and, therefore, the direction of the late depolarization forces will be to the right and anteriorly (Figure 4.7).

The diagnosis of right bundle branch block requires:

1. QRS of 0.12 seconds or more in duration.

2. Terminal S wave in lead I.

3. Terminal R^1 wave in lead V_1.

The significance of right bundle branch block:

1. Right bundle branch block may be seen in a heart which has a normal function, i.e. the appearance may be a normal variant.

2. Right bundle branch block may appear following an acute pulmonary embolus or in other conditions associated with dilatation of the right ventricle, e.g. atrial septal defect.

3. Occasionally the right bundle branch is involved in a myocardial infarct.

4. The many other less frequent causes of right bundle branch block include myocarditis, surgical section of the

right bundle when right ventriculotomy has been necessary, e.g. in the repair of a ventricular septal defect, and right bundle branch block may also be the first sign of degeneration of the entire conduction system of the heart.

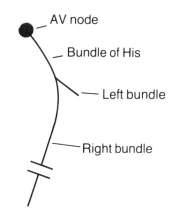

Figure 4.6.

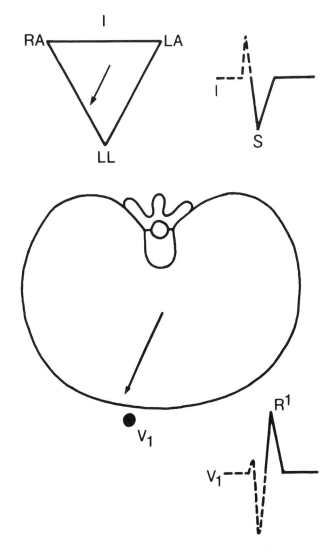

Figure 4.7. *Direction of terminal forces of depolarization in right bundle branch block. The effects of these terminal forces in leads I and V_1 are shown.*

Summary

Right ventricular hypertrophy is indicated by one or more of the following appearances:

1. Right axis deviation.

2. Ratio of R/S greater than 1 in lead V_1. Often accompanied by T inversion in V_1, V_2 and V_3.

3. Right axis deviation with RSR^1 in V_1.

4. T wave inversion in V_1, V_2, V_3 and V_4 which, in the absence of accompanying QRS changes, may indicate acute right ventricular dilation.

Electrocardiographic appearances in pulmonary embolism:

1. Electrocardiogram may be normal.

2. Right axis deviation with small P pulmonale.

3. Inverted T waves in V_1, V_2, V_3 and V_4.

4. RSR^1 in V_1.

5. Small Q waves in leads III and aVf.

Right bundle branch block. Three criteria are necessary for the diagnosis:

1. QRS complex 0.12 seconds or more in duration (three small squares or more).

2. Terminal S wave in lead I.

3. Terminal R^1 wave in lead V_1.

4. Electrocardiograms for Interpretation

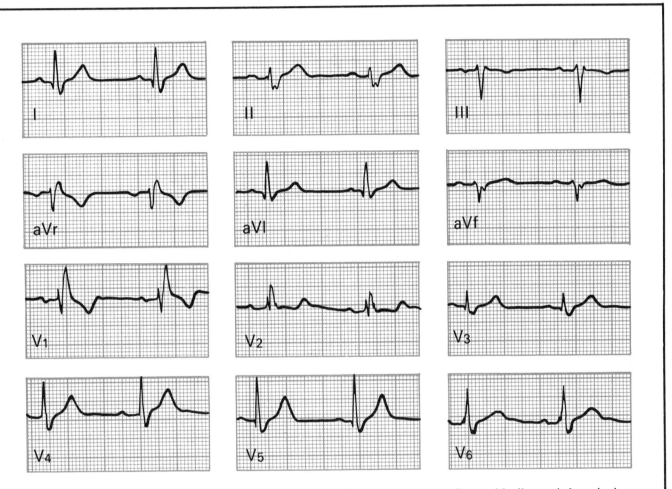

The QRS complexes are broad, in fact, the QRS duration in V_1 is four small squares, i.e. 0.16 seconds. Therefore, the diagnosis is bundle branch block.

Note the broad terminal S wave in lead I and the tall terminal R wave in V_1. The combination of a QRS greater than 0.12 seconds with terminal S in lead I and terminal R in V_1 makes the diagnosis right bundle branch block.

Furthermore, lead I is dominantly upright whereas leads II and III show dominantly negative QRS deflections. It was explained in Part 3 that this means left axis deviation.

The final electrocardiographic diagnosis here is sinus rhythm with a PR interval of 0.24 seconds, right bundle branch block and left axis deviation. (The long PR interval suggests poor conduction down the AV node and bundle of His, the right bundle branch block means no conduction down the right bundle, and the left axis deviation indicates that the conduction in the anterior division of the left bundle branch is impaired.)

The patient gives a history of blackouts and the electrocardiogram strongly suggests that the attacks are Stokes–Adams in nature due to episodes of complete heart block.

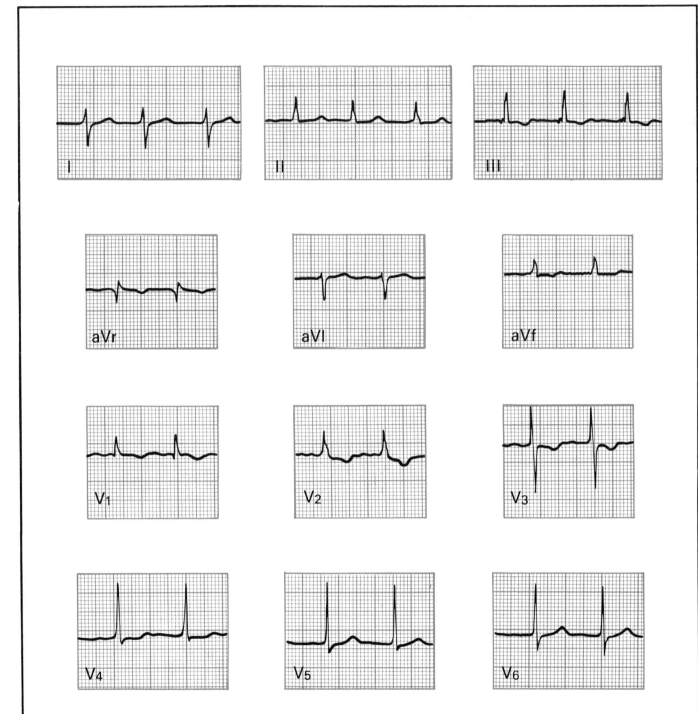

The QRS deflection is dominantly negative in lead I and positive in leads II and III. Therefore, there is right axis deviation.

V_1 shows a small Q wave and a tall R wave. The T waves are inverted in leads V_1, V_2 and V_3.

The diagnosis is right ventricular hypertrophy. No P waves are seen because the rhythm was atrial fibrillation.

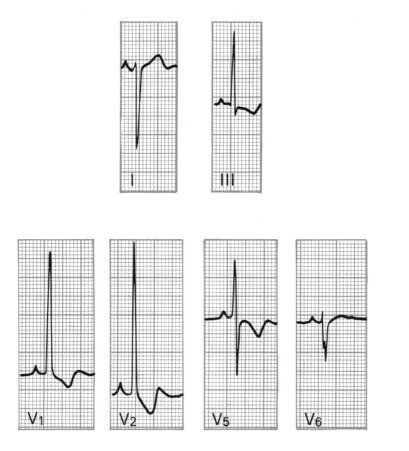

There is a deep S in lead I and tall R in lead III. Therefore, there is right axis deviation.

Huge R waves are present in precordial leads V_1 and V_2 and there is T wave inversion in all precordial leads up to and including V_5.

The electrocardiographic diagnosis is severe right ventricular hypertrophy and strain.

This electrocardiogram was taken from a boy with severe stenosis of the pulmonary valve. The stenosis was relieved at operation using cardiopulmonary bypass and subsequent electrocardiograms have shown a marked decrease in the right ventricular hypertrophy.

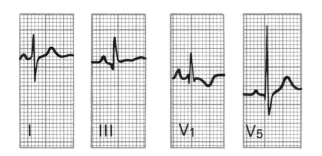

Right axis deviation is present.

Area of lead I is dominantly negative, area of lead III is positive. There is an RSR[1] complex visible in lead V_1.

This electrocardiogram was taken from a patient with an atrial septal defect. The electrocardiographic diagnosis of a large right ventricle was confirmed at surgery.

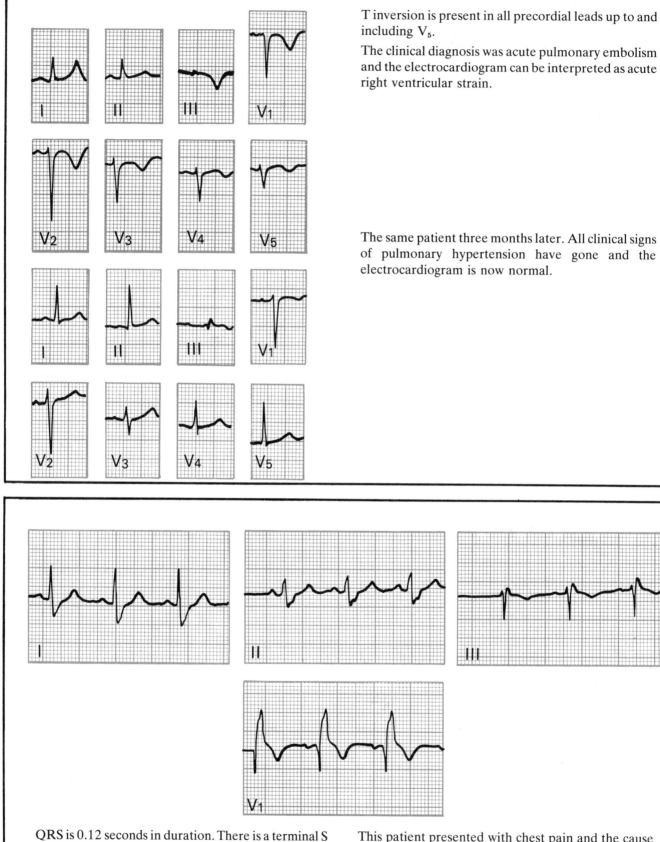

T inversion is present in all precordial leads up to and including V_5.

The clinical diagnosis was acute pulmonary embolism and the electrocardiogram can be interpreted as acute right ventricular strain.

The same patient three months later. All clinical signs of pulmonary hypertension have gone and the electrocardiogram is now normal.

QRS is 0.12 seconds in duration. There is a terminal S wave in lead I and a terminal R^1 wave in lead V_1, indicating complete right bundle branch block.

This patient presented with chest pain and the cause of the block was involvement of the right bundle branch by a myocardial infarct.

5. Myocardial Infarction

The diagnosis of myocardial infarction from the electrocardiogram depends upon the finding of pathological Q waves.

Myocardial infarction alters the initial forces of ventricular depolarization because the necrotic area of muscle does not undergo depolarization. This is the cause of the appearance of Q waves in the electrocardiogram.

In acute myocardial infarction the ST and T waves also undergo changes, but the diagnosis cannot be made with any degree of certainty from the electrocardiogram unless pathological Q waves are present.

Two criteria are necessary for the diagnosis of pathological Q waves:

1. The Q wave must be at least 0.04 seconds (one small square) in duration.

2. This Q wave is pathological only if it is present in leads that do not normally have Q waves.

Note. No mention has been made of the depth of the Q wave which is in fact relatively unimportant. If the Q wave is over 0.04 seconds in duration then it is pathological, irrespective of depth.

Normal Initial Ventricular Depolarization Forces

Figure 5.1 shows the direction of spread of the depolarization wave through the left ventricle during the first 0.04 seconds, indicated by the small arrows.

The average direction of spread during this time is the average of all the small arrows and is represented by the large arrow.

This average depolarization force will be seen in leads II and III as a current travelling towards the left leg and will be recorded as a positive deflection.

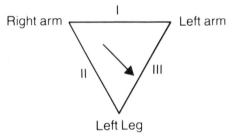

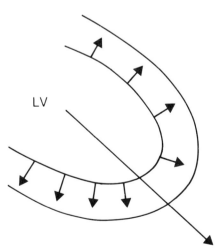

Figure 5.1.

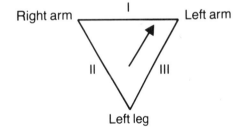

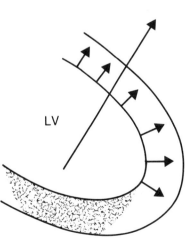

Figure 5.2.

Initial Ventricular Depolarization Forces in Myocardial Infarction

In Figure 5.2 the shaded area represents an infarct involving the inferior part of the left ventricular wall.

The necrotic area of muscle is not capable of undergoing depolarization in the normal manner and the large arrow indicates the average direction of spread of the remaining depolarization forces during the initial part of ventricular depolarization.

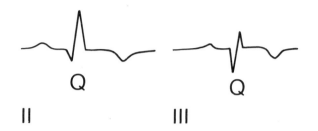

Figure 5.3.

Leads II and III now record a negative deflection during the initial ventricular depolarization (Figure 5.3).

An inferior myocardial infarct, then, is diagnosed from the appearance of Q waves in leads II and III.

Note. The older term 'posterior myocardial infarct' is also used for the electrocardiographic finding of Q waves in leads II and III. The term 'inferior myocardial infarct' is more accurate and is to be preferred.

We can now consider how the location of the infarct determines the leads in which pathological Q waves will appear.

Sites of Myocardial Infarction

Myocardial infarction affects the left ventricle. Three common sites recognized on the electrocardiogram are shown in Figure 5.4.

Inferior Myocardial Infarction

As explained, inferior myocardial infarction is characterized by pathological Q waves in leads II and III.

Anterior Myocardial Infarction

The anterior part of the left ventricle is infarcted. In Figure 5.5 the large arrow represents the direction of the depolarization wave which is travelling away from precordial leads V_1, V_2 and V_3.

An anterior infarct, then, is diagnosed from the appearance of Q waves in leads V_1, V_2 and V_3 (Figure 5.6).

Anterolateral Myocardial Infarct

Figure 5.7 shows a horizontal section through the chest and

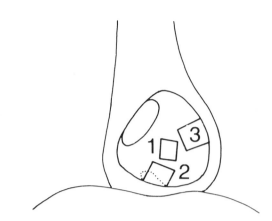

Figure 5.4. *Sites of myocardial infarction. 1 = anterior, 2 = inferior, 3 = anterolateral.*

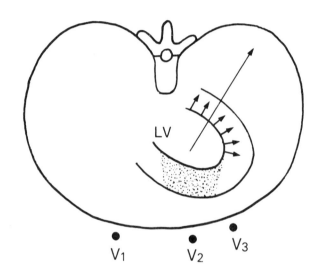

Figure 5.5. *Horizontal section through chest and heart to show anterior infarct. The forces are directed posteriorly away from the infarcted zone during the initial part of ventricular depolarization. Negative deflections are recorded in leads V_1, V_2 and V_3.*

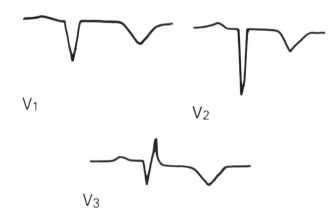

Figure 5.6.

...art to demonstrate anterolateral infarct.

...he initial wave of depolarization is travelling away from

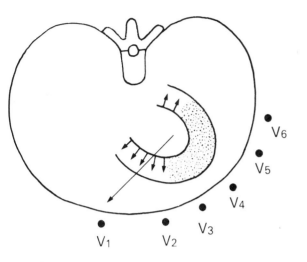

Figure 5.7.

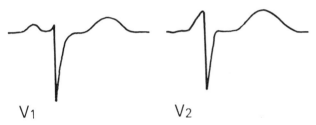

V₁ V₂

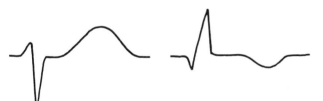

V₃ V₄

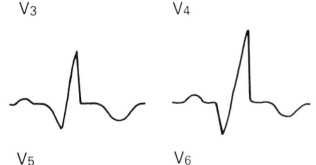

V₅ V₆

Figure 5.8.

...eads V₄, V₅ and V₆ and these leads will therefore show ...athological Q waves (Figure 5.8).

Strictly Posterior Myocardial Infarction

...When the infarct is confined to the posterior wall of the left ...entricle the diagnosis from the electrocardiogram can be ...ifficult.

A strictly posterior infarct will cause the initial ventricular depolarization forces to be directed anteriorly and will give large R waves in leads V₁, V₂ and V₃. These large R waves are not always recognizably abnormal and, furthermore, large R waves in V₁, V₂ and V₃ may be a normal finding which may occur in right ventricular hypertrophy and in chronic chest disease.

Usually the infarct also involves the lateral or inferior surface of the heart to some extent and gives changes in the appropriate leads.

The Evolution of the Electrocardiographic Changes in Myocardial Infarction

In myocardial infarction the electrocardiogram often undergoes a series of changes and this allows some approximations to be made about the dating of the infarct.

It is emphasized that the time scale is only approximate and frequently it is not possible to date the infarct from the electrocardiogram alone.

1. ST segment elevation occurs within minutes of the infarct. The elevated ST segment is usually straight (Figure 5.9) and this may help to distinguish myocardial infarction at this stage from acute pericarditis, which also gives rise to widespread ST segment elevation (Figure 5.10). In acute pericarditis the ST segment is usually bowed upwards.

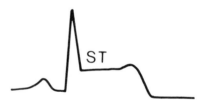

Figure 5.9.

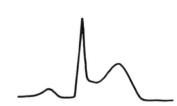

Figure 5.10. *Elevated ST segment due to acute pericarditis.*

2. Pathological Q waves appear (Figure 5.11), usually within hours of the onset of the infarct. Occasionally the Q waves appear 24 to 48 hours later. It is always worthwhile to repeat the electrocardiograms in a patient where a myocardial infarct is suspected but the initial electrocardiogram is normal or shows non-specific ST or T wave changes only.

3. The ST segment gradually becomes isoelectric again over the course of a few days to a few weeks and the T waves become inverted (Figure 5.12).

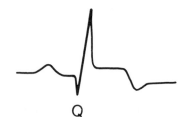

Q

Figure 5.11.

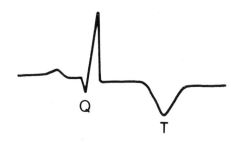

Q   T

Figure 5.12.

4. The final appearance of the electrocardiogram is variable. Often the T waves gradually resume their original upright shape and the Q waves may become narrow and less than 0.04 seconds in duration. These Q waves would not, therefore, be recognizably abnormal and the diagnosis of old myocardial infarction would not be justifiable from the final electrocardiogram alone.

Persistent ST segment elevation, three months or more after the onset of myocardial infarction, usually indicates that there is aneurysmal bulging of the left ventricular wall at the site of the old infarct.

Summary

Pathological Q waves in the electrocardiogram are the hallmarks of myocardial infarction.

ST and T changes in isolation do occur in some cases of myocardial infarction but are non-specific and leave the diagnosis in some doubt.

Pathological Q waves are recognized by:

1. Duration of 0.04 seconds (one small square) or more.

2. Occurrence in leads which do not normally show Q waves.

An anterior myocardial infarct has Q waves in precordial leads V_1, V_2 and V_3.

An inferior myocardial infarct has Q waves in leads II and III.

The earliest electrocardiographic sign of myocardial infarction is ST elevation, followed by the appearance of Q waves and of T inversion.

Some months after a myocardial infarct the electrocardiogram usually shows persistent Q waves, but occasionally may be within normal limits.

Persistent ST segment elevation months after myocardial infarction indicates left ventricular aneurysm formation.

5. Electrocardiograms for Interpretation

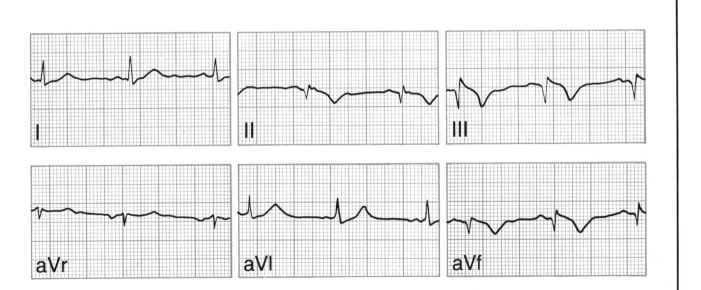

Pathological Q waves are present in leads II, III and aVf. The T wave is deeply inverted in these leads. This is inferior myocardial infarction.

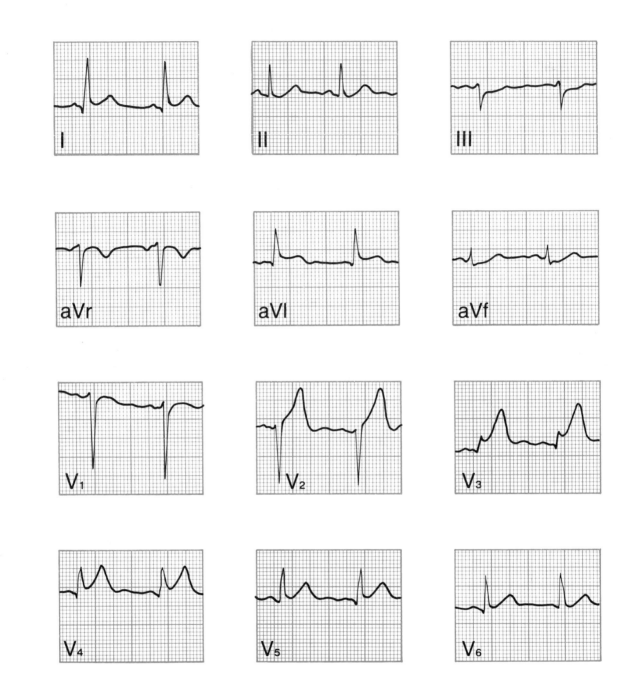

Normal QRS complexes.

There is definite ST segment elevation in leads I, aVl, V_2, V_3, V_4 and V_5. The patient had the clinical features of a myocardial infarct and this would be a probable diagnosis on this electrocardiogram.

There are no Q waves, however, and the diagnosis could not be made with great confidence from this electrocardiogram alone.

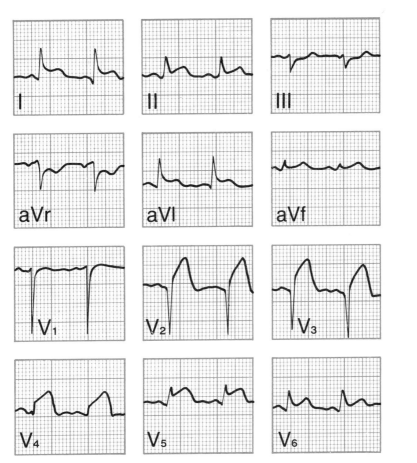

Electrocardiogram from the same patient recorded 24 hours later. There are now pathological Q waves in leads V_2, V_3 and V_4. This second tracing is therefore very helpful and confirms the diagnosis of anterior myocardial infarction.

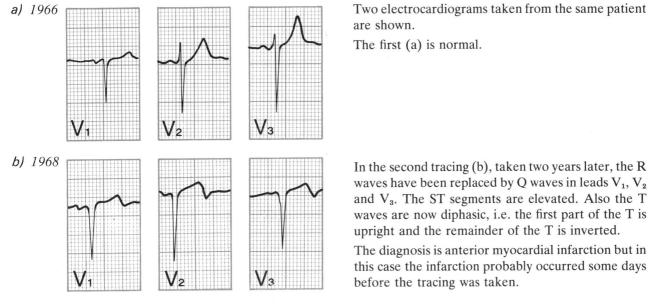

a) 1966

b) 1968

Two electrocardiograms taken from the same patient are shown.

The first (a) is normal.

In the second tracing (b), taken two years later, the R waves have been replaced by Q waves in leads V_1, V_2 and V_3. The ST segments are elevated. Also the T waves are now diphasic, i.e. the first part of the T is upright and the remainder of the T is inverted.

The diagnosis is anterior myocardial infarction but in this case the infarction probably occurred some days before the tracing was taken.

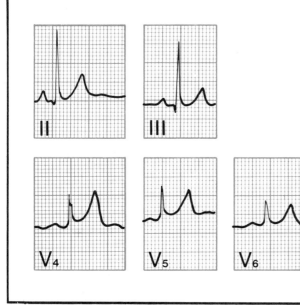

Widespread ST segment elevation.

The shape of the ST segments—concave upwards—suggests that the diagnosis here is acute pericarditis and this proved to be correct.

However, in acute early myocardial infarction widespread ST segment elevation is also seen and the differential diagnosis is best made from other clinical features and from repeated ECGs rather than by reliance on the exact shape of the ST segments.

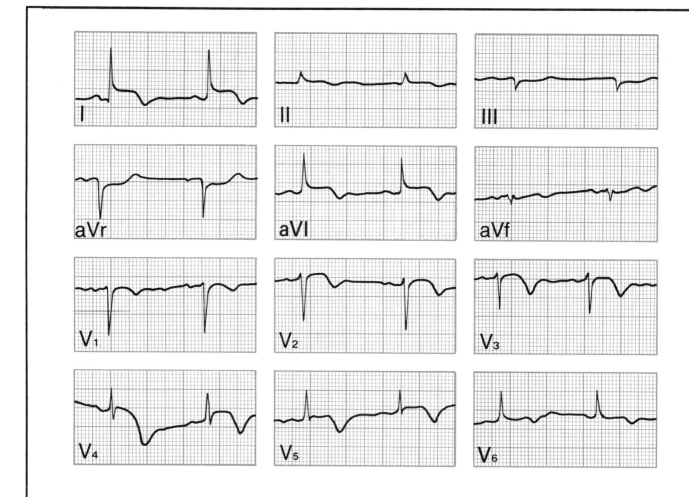

ST segment elevation in leads I and aVl with T wave inversion in V_2 to V_6. Note the flat contour of the elevated ST segment.

Appearances suggest anterolateral myocardial infarction and this was the diagnosis in this patient.

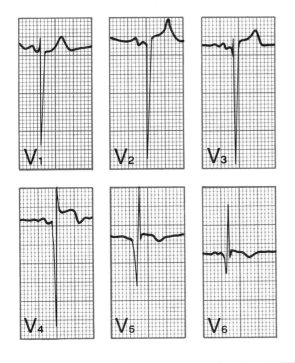

Q waves are present in leads V_4, V_5 and V_6, the ST segment is elevated in those leads and the T wave is inverted.

Recent anterolateral myocardial infarction is a possible diagnosis but the history indicates that a myocardial infarction occurred six months before the recording of this ECG and that many ECGs over a period of some months have shown persistent ST segment elevation.

The diagnosis of left ventricular aneurysm following myocardial infarction was made and the aneurysm was resected at operation with considerable improvement in the patient's signs and symptoms of cardiac failure.

6. The ST Segment

The ST segment of the electrocardiogram (Figure 6.1) represents the period from the completion of ventricular depolarization (end of QRS) to the beginning of ventricular repolarization (beginning of T wave).

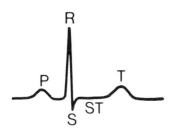

Figure 6.1.

The ST segment is normally isoelectric, i.e. at the base line. Every tracing should be carefully examined for any ST displacement above or below the base line.

Abnormalities of the ST segment are often the only electrocardiographic sign of disease and the smallest shift in the ST segment must be explained. In general, the normal ST segment is not displaced more than 0.5 mm except in precordial leads V_1 and V_2 where it may exceed this slightly.

Unfortunately, although ST segment variation may be an important indication of disease, there are several diseases and at least one normal condition where the ST segment is affected.

ST abnormalities on the electrocardiogram alone are rarely diagnostic and the electrocardiogram can be interpreted only when the symptoms and signs are also available.

The exact pattern of ST segment abnormality tends to vary according to the underlying condition and may provide some help in reaching the correct diagnosis.

The various conditions causing ST abnormalities will now be considered.

Subendocardial Ischaemia

Ischaemia of the subendocardial region occurs in acute coronary insufficiency and in angina pectoris.

The terminal branches of the coronary arteries supply the subendocardial region of the heart muscle and when there is insufficient coronary blood flow the subendocardial region suffers first.

The electrocardiogram shows ST segment depression, often widespread, but particularly evident in precordial leads V_4, V_5 and V_6.

Note the characteristic features (Figure 6.2):

1. The junction of the ST segment with the QRS complex is depressed well below the isoelectric line.

2. The ST segment is straight and horizontal.

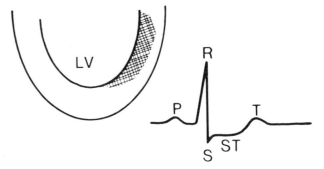

Figure 6.2.

Epicardial Injury

Widespread ST segment elevation is the first electrocardiographic abnormality in acute myocardial infarction and was described in Part 5. ST elevation (Figure 6.3) occurs in leads over the site of the infarct and the ST segment is usually straight and horizontal. Q waves appear soon after the ST changes and the ST segment returns to the base line within days or weeks of the myocardial infarct.

Persistent elevation months after the infarct usually indicates aneurysm formation of the left ventricle at the site of the infarct.

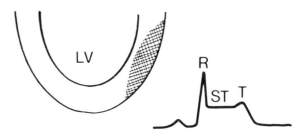

Figure 6.3.

Epicardial injury also occurs in acute pericarditis and is probably responsible for the widespread ST elevation of this condition. In acute pericarditis the ST segment retains a concave upwards configuration (Figure 6.4) and this appearance may help in distinguishing the electrocardiogram of acute pericarditis from that of myocardial infarction.

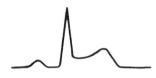

Figure 6.4.

Q waves do not appear at any time during acute pericarditis.

Digitalis Effect

Digitalis causes a sagging depression of the ST segment (Figure 6.5), usually with little or no depression in the QRS–ST junction.

Such shifts, however, may appear and the differential diagnosis between a digitalis effect and subendocardial ischaemia may be difficult or impossible.

Great caution is necessary before attributing an ST segment depression to subendocardial ischaemia if the patient is receiving, or has recently received, digitalis.

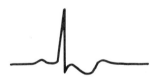

Figure 6.5.

Left Ventricular Hypertrophy

ST segment depression in association with large QRS voltages (Figure 6.6) indicates left ventricular hypertrophy of considerable severity and has been described in Part 2.

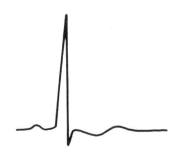

Figure 6.6.

Normal Variant of ST in Young Adults

In normal young adults very large upright T waves in precordial leads V_4, V_5 and V_6 are not unusual.

ST elevation commonly accompanies the tall T waves (Figure 6.7), occurs in the same leads as the tall T waves and is of no pathological significance.

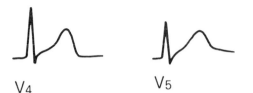

Figure 6.7.

This normal variant may be distinguished from acute pericarditis by the following features:

1. The T waves are normal in size or small in acute pericarditis.

2. The ST segment returns to the base line within a few weeks at most in acute pericarditis.

3. During mild exercise the electrocardiogram will show persistent ST elevation in acute pericarditis, but the ST segment becomes isoelectric when the ST elevation is a normal variant.

Metabolic Abnormalities

Potassium deficiency is the commonest of these in clinical practice.

A low serum potassium results in a low T wave with ST segment depression.

These changes quickly revert to normal when potassium is given.

The Electrocardiogram in Angina Pectoris

It is most important to note that the electrocardiogram is commonly normal in patients with angina pectoris.

The diagnosis of angina pectoris is made from the history and if this is typical then a normal electrocardiogram will not influence the diagnosis.

When an electrocardiogram is abnormal the most characteristic feature of angina pectoris is a flat depression of the ST segment in leads V_4, V_5 and V_6, indicating subendocardial ischaemia.

In a considerable proportion of patients with myocardial ischaemia caused by coronary arterial disease some abnormality of the electrocardiogram will appear during or immediately after exercise.

If, after a full history and physical examination, there is reasonable doubt of the diagnosis an electrocardiogram taken during or after carefully controlled exercise may be helpful.

Summary

Any deviation of the ST segment above or below the isoelectric line should be regarded with suspicion.

Causes of ST segment depression:

1. *Subendocardial ischaemia.* ST segment is straight. QRS–ST junction is depressed below the base line.

2. *Digitalis effect.* ST segment sags. QRS–ST junction is not usually depressed.

3. *Left ventricular hypertrophy.* QRS complexes are of abnormally large voltage. ST segment is not straight but tends to go down and up, presenting a wave-like appearance.

4. *Metabolic abnormalities.* Low serum potassium causes ST depression and low amplitude T waves. These revert quickly to normal when the serum potassium is restored to normal levels.

Causes of ST segment elevation:

1. *Acute myocardial infarction.* ST segment is straight. Usually pathological Q waves soon appear.

2. *Acute pericarditis.* ST segment is concave upwards. Pathological Q waves do not appear.

3. *Normal variant.* Occurs in association with tall T waves. Usually found in symptom-free young adults.

The electrocardiogram in angina pectoris:

1. Commonly normal when recorded with the patient at rest.

2. The most characteristic abnormality is a straight ST segment depression, indicating subendocardial ischaemia, which is occasionally found at rest but more commonly appears only during or after exercise.

6. Electrocardiograms for Interpretation

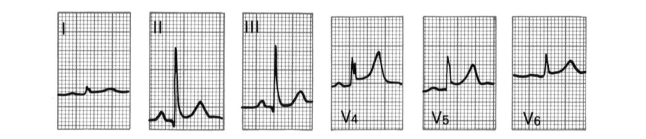

ST segment elevation is widespread, the ST segment being concave upwards.

In this patient the ST changes were caused by acute pericarditis.

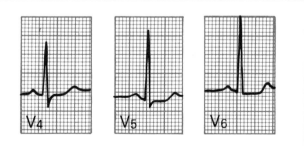

There is slight but definite ST segment depression in V₅ and V₆.

This degree of depression is significant, particularly, as in this case, when the ST segment is straight.

The diagnosis here was angina pectoris.

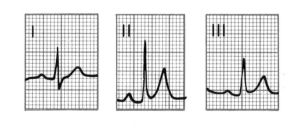

ST segment elevated and concave upwards, with tall T waves.

Comparing this with the previous example it is obvious that this normal variant can readily be confused with acute pericarditis if a single electrocardiogram is the only information available.

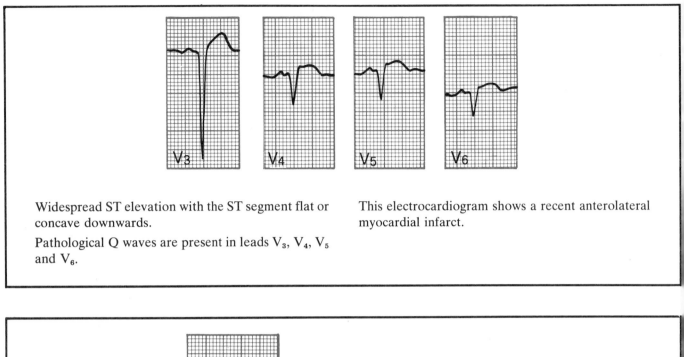

Widespread ST elevation with the ST segment flat or concave downwards.

Pathological Q waves are present in leads V_3, V_4, V_5 and V_6.

This electrocardiogram shows a recent anterolateral myocardial infarct.

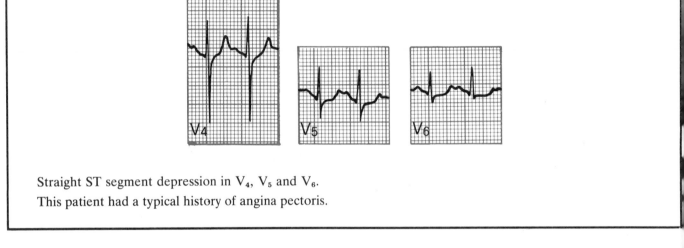

Straight ST segment depression in V_4, V_5 and V_6.

This patient had a typical history of angina pectoris.

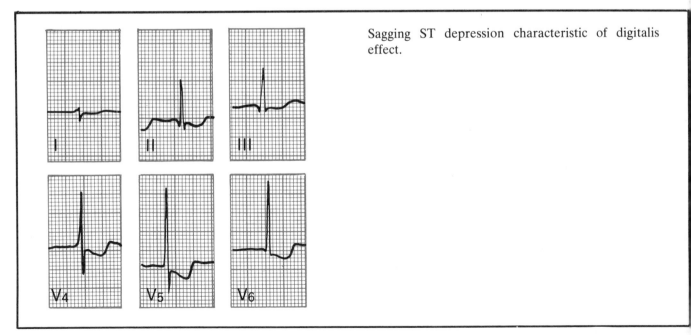

Sagging ST depression characteristic of digitalis effect.

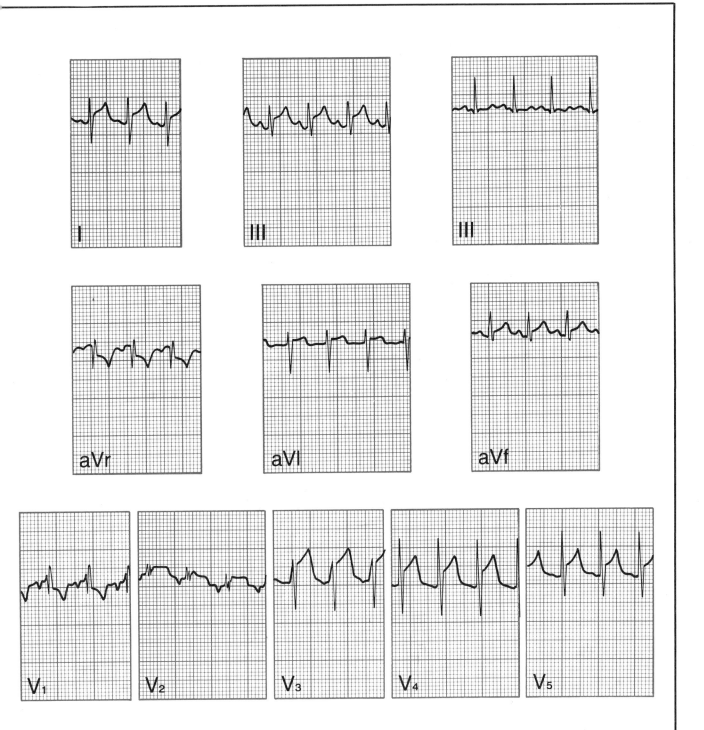

The electrocardiogram of a man aged 23, six days after surgery for closure of an atrial septal defect.

There is widespread ST segment elevation, particularly obvious in leads I, II, V_2, V_3, V_4 and V_5.

These were the changes of acute pericarditis and this patient required pericardial drainage because of tamponade. He then made a complete recovery.

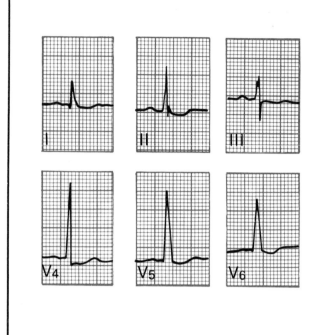

Sagging ST depression in leads II, III, V₄, V₅ and V₆.
The shape of ST is characteristic of a digitalis effect.

This patient was in fact receiving digoxin 0.25 mg t.d.s.

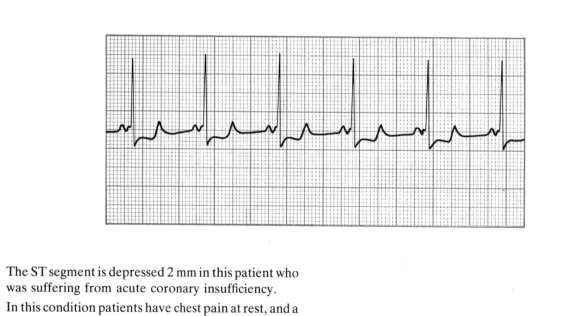

The ST segment is depressed 2 mm in this patient who was suffering from acute coronary insufficiency.

In this condition patients have chest pain at rest, and a proportion later develop myocardial infarction.

7. The Exercise Test for Ischaemic Heart Disease

The electrocardiogram recorded at rest is normal in over 50 per cent of patients suffering from classic angina pectoris. When the history is typical—pressure in the centre of the chest related to effort such as walking after meals or walking in the cold, lasting two to three minutes and relieved immediately by glyceryl trinitrate—the diagnosis is angina pectoris and should be made without further special electrocardiographic tests.

A normal electrocardiogram is not unusual in such a case.

The electrocardiogram recorded during or immediately after exercise is required in two main clinical situations:

. In patients with a history of pain or chest discomfort not typical for angina pectoris with a normal resting electrocardiogram. If ischaemic heart disease is suspected an exercise electrocardiogram may prove useful in this situation.

. For the diagnosis of entirely asymptomatic coronary arterial disease, e.g. in airline pilots, bus and train drivers.

Methods of Recording an Exercise Electrocardiogram

The master two-step test is a well-known method. The patient walks up and down two steps, each nine inches in height for a prescribed number of times, determined by age, sex and weight, all within a three-minute period. The electrocardiogram is recorded immediately after exercise, two minutes later and finally six minutes after completion of the exercise. Leads V_4, V_5, V_6, V_3 and standard lead II are recorded on each occasion, and usually in that order.

A second popular non-standardized method is to prescribe a number of flights of stairs to be walked up, the number of flights depending on the physician's assessment of the patient's accustomed level of exercise. Again the electrocardiogram should be recorded immediately after exertion, and at two and six minutes following their exercise.

In the cardiac laboratory exercise testing is performed using a treadmill or a bicycle ergometer. The heart rate can be used as a guide to the severity of the exertion and the work load is increased every three minutes until maximal exertion, or such level of exertion as has been previously determined, is reached. The electrocardiogram is recorded continuously with careful monitoring of the patient's general condition, blood pressure and respiration.

Special Precautions

1. The exercise test should be performed only by a physician.

2. A careful history is taken immediately before the test. If there have been any bouts of severe pain in the last week an impending myocardial infarction is possible and the test should be cancelled.

3. A full electrocardiogram is recorded immediately before the test and must be completely normal.

4. The patient is warned that he must stop immediately if he experiences pain or pressure in the chest, arms or neck.

Interpretation of the Exercise Electrocardiogram

This is by no means easy, even after considerable experience. In the presence of coronary artery disease 'ischaemic' depression of the ST segment is the most usual and also the most reliable finding.

This depression is often at its maximum in the electrocardiogram recorded immediately after exertion but may appear only some minutes later.

The need to record the electrocardiogram again at two and six minutes after exercise is emphasized. Ideally, the electrocardiogram should be monitored during exercise and it is claimed that in some patients abnormalities are present only during this time.

A normal exercise electrocardiogram does not exclude the possibility of coronary artery disease, even when the test has been performed in the laboratory under ideal conditions and to a high grade of exertion. (The appearance of a normal ST segment before exercise is shown in Figure 7.1.)

Findings in the Exercise Electrocardiogram Indicating Ischaemic Heart Disease

Ischaemic Depression of the ST Segment

The ST segment is depressed 1 mm or more.

The ST segment is horizontal or, in some cases, sags downwards to the beginning of the T wave (Figure 7.2).

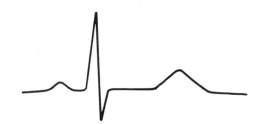

Figure 7.1. *V₄ before exercise. Normal.*

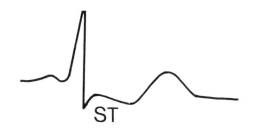

Figure 7.2. *a) V₄ immediately after exercise. Sagging depression of ST.*

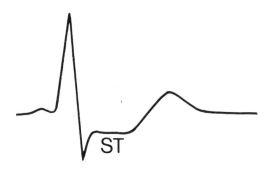

b) V₄ immediately after exercise. Horizontal depression of ST.

A depression of less than 1 mm in the absence of a typical history of ischaemic heart disease is regarded as equivocal.

Elevation of the ST Segment

It is unusual for ST segment elevation to occur after exercise in a patient with a normal pre-exercise electrocardiogram. When seen, however, it indicates ischaemic heart disease.

The Appearance of Left Bundle Branch Block

Left bundle branch block is characterized by a QRS complex width of more than 0.12 seconds with tiny or more usually absent Q waves in leads I, V₅ and V₆ and tiny or absent R waves in precordial lead V₁ (Figure 7.3).

The transient appearance of left bundle branch block after exercise may indicate an abnormal coronary arterial system.

The Occurrence of an Arrhythmia

Rarely, a very transient ventricular tachycardia (Figure 7.4) is seen at the completion of exercise and indicate serious disease.

Complete heart block (Figure 7.5) at the end of the exercise may indicate coronary artery disease.

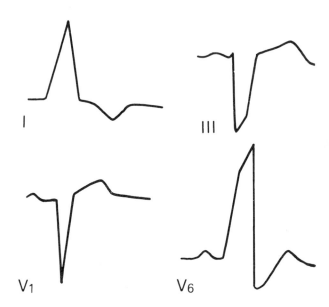

Figure 7.3. *Left bundle branch block after exercise.*

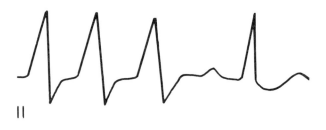

Figure 7.4. *Short episode of ventricular tachycardia after exercise. The last ventricular complex shows normal rhythm.*

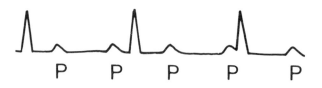

Figure 7.5. *Complete heart block.*

Multifocal ventricular premature contractions (Figure 7.6) are frequently seen at the end of exercise and indicate serious disease.

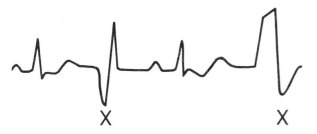

Figure 7.6. *Lead II after exercise in a patient with ischaemic heart disease. Two ventricular extrasystoles, marked X, can be seen. They differ from one another in configuration indicating that there is more than one ectopic focus in the ventricles.*

Atrial tachycardia and atrial fibrillation are uncommon.

All these arrhythmias are regarded as indicating ischaemic heart disease when they appear during or immediately after the exercise test.

T wave Changes

Minor T wave changes are practically the rule during and after exercise and do not indicate disease.

However, if an upright T wave of at least 1.5 mm becomes inverted to at least the same amount this is regarded as abnormal and indicative of ischaemic heart disease.

U wave Changes

The U wave on the electrocardiogram is usually of little or no clinical significance.

The normal U wave is an additional deflection after the T wave and, when present, is most conspicuous in precordial leads V_3, V_4, V_5 and V_6.

U waves tend to be prominent when the blood potassium is low.

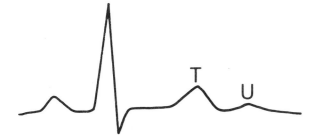

Figure 7.7. *Lead V_4. The normal U wave, when present, is upright.*

The normal U waves are upright in precordial leads V_4 (Figure 7.7), V_5 and V_6, and inversion of the U waves in these leads after exercise is considered to indicate coronary arterial disease.

Junctional Depression: A Common Normal Finding after Exercise

This must not be confused with the changes of ischaemic heart disease.

The junction between the QRS and the beginning of the ST segment is called the J point.

After exercise the J point may normally be well below the base line (Figure 7.8). This normal junctional depression is the result of several factors.

Probably the most important of these is the influence of the atrial repolarization (Ta) wave (Figure 7.9). Usually the wave of atrial repolarization is completely hidden in the QRS complex.

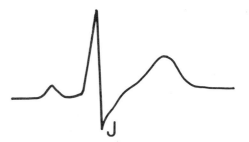

Figure 7.8. *Junctional depression. Not ischaemic.*

After exercise the PR interval is shortened and the atrial repolarization wave is increased in magnitude.

The effect of this large repolarization wave is to depress the J point (Figure 7.10).

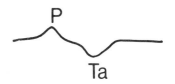

Figure 7.9. *Atrial depolarization, P wave, is followed by atrial repolarization, the Ta wave.*

The important feature differentiating this normal junctional depression from the ischaemic ST change is the appearance of the ST segment.

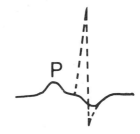

Figure 7.10. *The interrupted line represents ventricular depolarization. Junctional depression caused by the atrial T wave is shown.*

In normal subjects the ST segment slopes rapidly upwards from the J point to the T wave.

In ischaemic heart disease the ST segment is horizontal or may even sag downwards after the J point.

Summary

An electrocardiogram recorded after exercise is useful in the diagnosis of ischaemic heart disease when the resting electrocardiogram is normal. Essential steps in recording the exercise electrocardiogram include:

1. The presence of a physician throughout the test.

2. A completely normal electrocardiogram immediately before exercise begins.

3. No history of chest pain suggesting a recent myocardial infarct.

4. Immediate termination of exercise if the patient develops pain or discomfort.

The test is regarded as positive if the electrocardiogram shows one or more of the following features after exercise:

1. Ischaemic ST segment depression.

2. Bursts of ventricular extrasytoles or other serious arrhythmias.

3. ST segment elevation.

4. Gross changes in the T waves.

5. The appearance of left bundle branch block.

Ischaemic ST segment depression is the most usual and most important of these changes.

In fact, ST depression is nearly always found when any of the other positive features are present.

Great care must be taken to distinguish junctional depression, a common normal appearance after exercise, from ischaemic ST segment depression.

The differentiation is made from the subsequent behaviour of the ST segment.

In myocardial ischaemia the ST segment runs horizontally or even slopes downwards to the beginning of the T wave.

7. Electrocardiograms for Interpretation

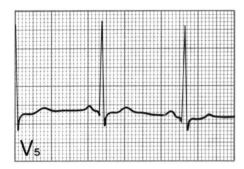

Before exercise.

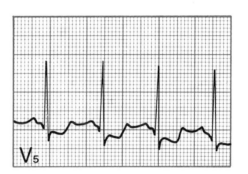

Immediately after exercise.

This patient gave a history of chest pain but the pain bore little relation to exercise and the electrocardiogram recorded at rest was normal.

An exercise test was performed and the tracings show V_5 within normal limits before exercise but grossly abnormal immediately after exercise.

The ST segment is depressed below the base line and slopes downward to the beginning of the T wave.

This is a classically positive exercise test. The patient has ischaemic heart disease.

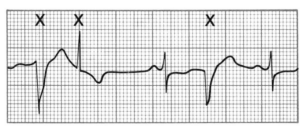

Lead II, recorded immediately after exercise. Ventricular extrasystoles (X) have appeared.

Note that the extrasystoles have varying shapes, proving that they arise from more than one focus in the ventricles.

This is a positive exercise test. The patient has ischaemic heart disease and is in danger of developing ventricular fibrillation.

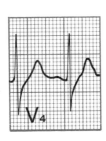

The J point is depressed, but thereafter the ST segment slopes upwards steeply to the T wave.

This lead was recorded immediately after exercise and is a common normal finding.

There is no evidence of ischaemic heart disease from this test.

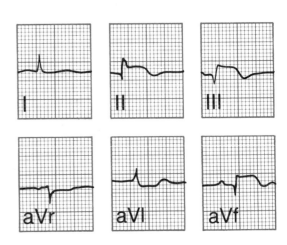

This patient was referred for an exercise test to help in the diagnosis of chest pain.

The electrocardiogram recorded at rest is shown.

The exercise test must not be performed because this electrocardiogram shows an acute posterior myocardial infarction.

Exercise would be dangerous and is entirely unnecessary.

The diagnosis is obvious.

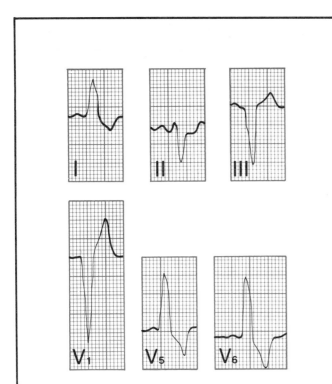

The QRS complexes are wide and exceed 0.12 seconds in duration. In fact, they measure 0.16 seconds (four small squares).

There are no Q waves in leads I, V_5 or V_6, and no R wave in lead V_1.

This is left bundle branch block. When this appears during or after exercise, coronary artery disease may be present.

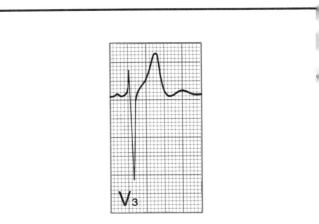

QRS complex followed by a large T wave which in turn is followed by a smaller positive wave.

This small positive wave is a normal U wave. Very large U waves may be evidence of a low blood potassium.

Occasionally, after an exercise test, the U waves become inverted and evidence exists to suggest that this indicates myocardial ischaemia.

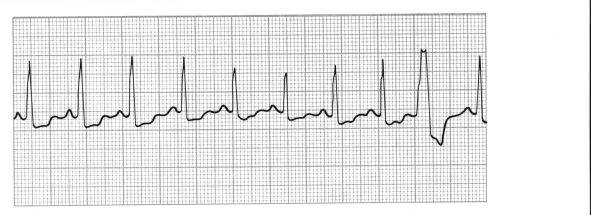

A positive exercise test.

ST depression is very obvious and there is one ventricular extrasystole.

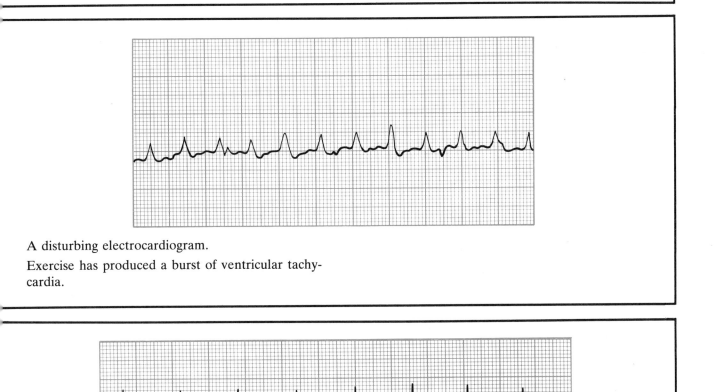

A disturbing electrocardiogram.

Exercise has produced a burst of ventricular tachycardia.

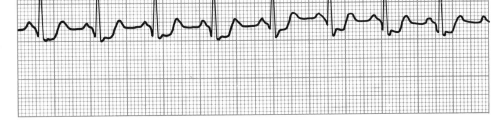

A positive exercise test.

The exercise was not strenuous, the heart rate reaching 100 beats per minute. The ST segment is depressed 2 mm, and the ST depression in this patient is of the typical horizontal shape of myocardial ischaemia.

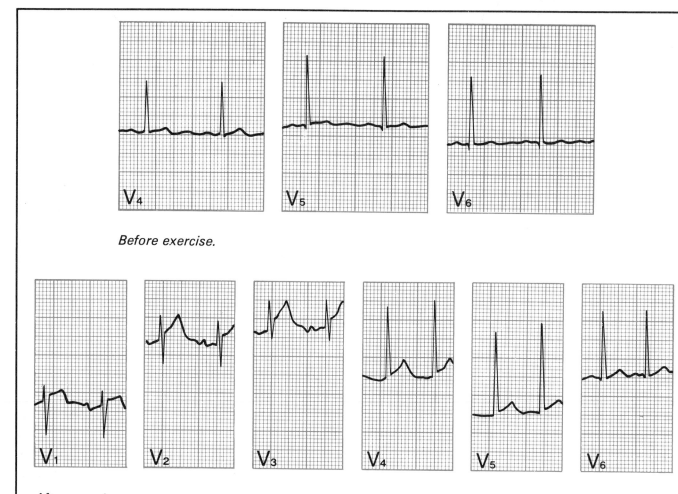

Before exercise.

After exercise.

An unusual finding on exercise.

Before the exercise test V_4, V_5 and V_6 are seen to be within normal limits.

After exercise there is ST segment elevation in precordial leads V_1 to V_5.

This is an example of Prinzmetal's angina. Often these patients have obstruction of the left main coronary artery and the attacks of angina tend to bear little relation to exertion.

8. The T wave

Figure 8.1.

The Normal T wave

The T wave represents repolarization of the ventricles and occurs in the electrocardiogram immediately after the ST segment.

The sequence of ventricular electrical activity throughout the cardiac cycle is as follows:

1. Ventricular depolarization—a fast process seen on the electrocardiogram as rapid QRS deflections.

2. A phase of electrical inactivity at the end of ventricular depolarization, seen as the flat isoelectric ST segment.

3. A phase of ventricular repolarization as the myocardial cells slowly recover their original charge and the T wave is written on the electrocardiogram.

Shape of the T wave

The normal T wave is slightly asymmetric (Figure 8.1).

The initial upward deflection rises slowly to the peak but the descending limb falls more steeply back to the base line (Figure 8.2).

Direction of the T wave

If repolarization of the ventricles followed the same pathway as ventricular depolarization the T wave would be equal in magnitude but of opposite direction to the QRS complex.

The normal T wave, however, is usually in the same direction as the QRS complex.

In the leads with mainly positive QRS complexes the T waves are usually upright, and when the QRS complex is

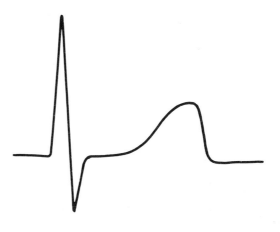

Figure 8.2. *Magnified electrocardiogram to show the more gradual rising limb of the T wave.*

mainly negative the T waves are negative, i.e. below the base line.

It is therefore apparent that in the normal heart repolarization does not take the same pathway as depolarization.

A useful rule to remember is that in the adult, in leads I and II the T wave is upright, and in the precordial leads the T wave becomes upright in either V_1 or V_2. Thereafter, it steadily gains in amplitude being tallest in leads V_5 and V_6 (Figure 8.3).

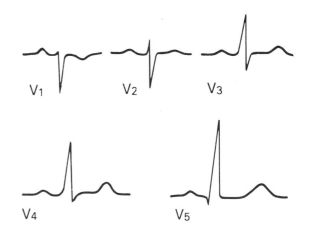

Figure 8.3.

Amplitude of the T wave

The height of the T wave varies considerably between patients, and even in the same patient there may be a normal day to day fluctuation in the size of the T wave.

No precise figures can be given for the upper and lower limits of the T wave in each lead.

Very tall T waves, and the opposite extreme almost flat T waves, may be of help in the diagnosis but a change in the *direction* of the wave from upright to negative or vice versa is a much more significant finding.

Causes of T wave Abnormalities

Ventricular repolarization is a process sensitive to a large number of physiological as well as pathological influences.

Slight fluctuations from day to day in the size of the T wave in the individual patient are normal, and exercise, sleep, the ingestion of a large meal and other normal activities may all produce some T wave changes.

Of the many abnormalities producing T wave changes the following list will help to emphasize that the T wave is affected by a wide variety of influences and that in the electrocardiogram T wave changes alone must be regarded as non-specific.

Causes of T abnormality include:

Anaemia, severe infections, hepatitis, acidosis, shock, anoxia, myxoedema, drugs, e.g. digitalis, potassium, emetine, etc.

Diseases commonly resulting in T wave abnormalities will now be considered and any particular features on the electrocardiogram which might favour one particular diagnosis will be indicated.

Myocardial Ischaemia and Myocardial Infarction

The normal direction of the repolarization wave is downward and to the left.

The T wave vector makes a narrow angle with the normal QRS vector (Figure 8.4).

When the effect of a T wave force of this direction is studied in the usual way—using the equilateral triangle and remembering that a force travelling towards the left leg is recorded as positive in leads II and III (Figure 8.5), and that a force travelling towards the left arm is recorded as positive in lead I—a positive deflection will be recorded in all three limb leads.

In the presence of severe ischaemia or infarction the affected area of the myocardium gives no repolarization forces and the T forces from the uninvolved regions of the ventricle now have the effect of making the T wave point away from the ischaemic zone (Figure 8.6).

When this new T force is plotted on the standard leads it can

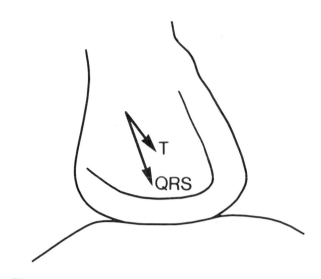

Figure 8.4.

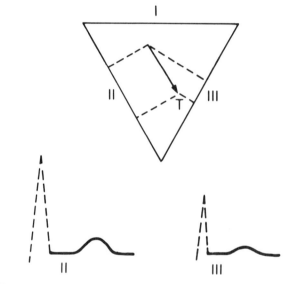

Figure 8.5.

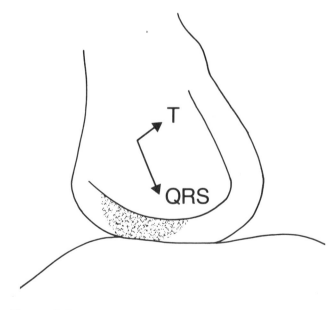

Figure 8.6.

60

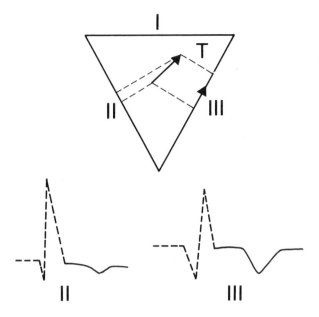

Figure 8.7.

...e seen that a localized area of inferior myocardial ischaemia or infarction causes negative T waves in leads II and III (Figure 8.7).

Any other localized area of myocardial injury may similarly produce a change in the direction of the T wave force and hence bring about alterations in the T waves, the leads affected depending upon the area involved.

In myocardial infarction the T waves are usually deep and symmetrical. The diagnosis has a firm basis if there are also pathological Q waves.

Myocardial infarction may certainly be present when localized T wave inversion is the sole electrocardiographic abnormality, but the diagnosis then requires confirmation from such features as a history of chest pain and a rise in serum transaminases.

Left Ventricular Ischaemia

Generalized ischaemia of the left ventricle causes the T wave forces to point away from this chamber.

The left ventricle lies posteriorly and in left ventricular ischaemia the T forces come to point anteriorly and are recorded as tall T waves in the anterior precordial leads V_1, V_2 and V_3 (Figure 8.8), whereas in leads V_4, V_5 and V_6 the T wave becomes progressively more flat.

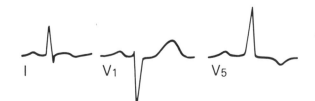

Figure 8.8.

In the limb leads the new direction of the T force results in low amplitude or inverted T waves in lead I.

Pericarditis

Early pericarditis, with the ensuing epicardial injury, is recognized on the electrocardiogram by widespread ST segment elevation involving most leads.

Later, as the ST segment becomes isoelectric, widespread T inversion develops in the precordial and limb leads.

The widespread nature of the T abnormalities serves to distinguish this condition from the localized T inversion of ischaemia or infarction, but many mistakes will be made if the differential diagnosis is made from the electrocardiogram in isolation from the other clinical and laboratory data.

Acute Right Ventricular Strain

Sudden obstruction of the pulmonary artery by a pulmonary embolus causes dilatation of the right ventricle.

The T wave forces change in direction to point away from the affected right ventricle.

Negative T waves may appear in the anterior precordial leads V_1, V_2 and V_3 and also in leads II, III and aVf in the first few hours following an acute pulmonary embolism.

Right Ventricular Hypertrophy

Right ventricular hypertrophy caused by an increased pressure load such as pulmonary valve stenosis or pulmonary hypertension was described in Part 4.

The QRS complexes are altered: there is right axis deviation accompanied by tall R waves in precordial leads V_1 and V_2.

The forces of repolarization may also be affected in the right ventricle and the result is negative T waves in leads V_1 and V_2.

Considerable hypertrophy is present before T wave changes become obvious.

Some guide to the severity of the hypertrophy may thus be obtained from the electrocardiogram, the presence of T wave changes indicating more advanced hypertrophy.

Summary

The T wave represents ventricular repolarization. This process is disturbed by a wide variety of influences, including some physiological processes.

T wave changes on the electrocardiogram are non-specific in the sense that a definite diagnosis should not be made on the basis of the electrocardiogram alone.

The normal T wave:

1. Upright in those leads having an upright QRS complex.

2. In the adult, may be inverted in lead V_1 and occasionally

in lead V_2.

3. Should gradually increase in height from right to left across the precordium, being upright and tallest in leads V_5 and V_6.

Generalized left ventricular ischaemia:
Flattening of the T waves in leads I, V_5 and V_6.

Localized area of left ventricular ischaemia or infarction:
The T wave points away from the affected region.

Inferior infarct:
T inversion in leads II, III, and aVf.

Lateral infarct:
T inversion in leads I, aVl, V_5 and V_6.

Pericarditis in the later stages of the disease:
Widespread T inversion involving most leads.

Acute right ventricular strain:
T inversion in leads V_1, V_2 and V_3 accompanied by right axis deviation.

Right ventricular hypertrophy:
T inversion in V_1, V_2 and V_3 accompanied by tall R waves in these leads and right axis deviation.

8. Electrocardiograms for Interpretation

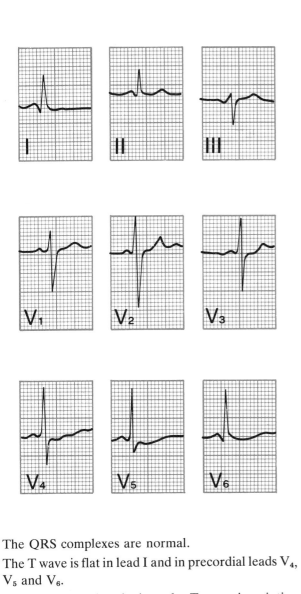

The QRS complexes are normal.

The T wave is flat in lead I and in precordial leads V_4, V_5 and V_6.

This is abnormal and, since the T wave is pointing away from the left ventricle, the most likely diagnosis is left ventricular ischaemia.

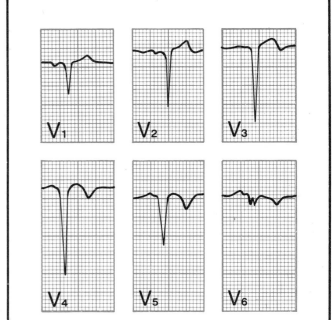

Q waves are present in all precordial leads and the T waves are inverted in leads V_4, V_5 and V_6.

This represents an extensive anterolateral myocardial infarct.

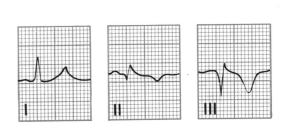

Deep symmetrical T wave inversion is present in leads II and III. A pathological Q wave is seen in lead III and a small Q in lead II.

This is an inferior myocardial infarct.

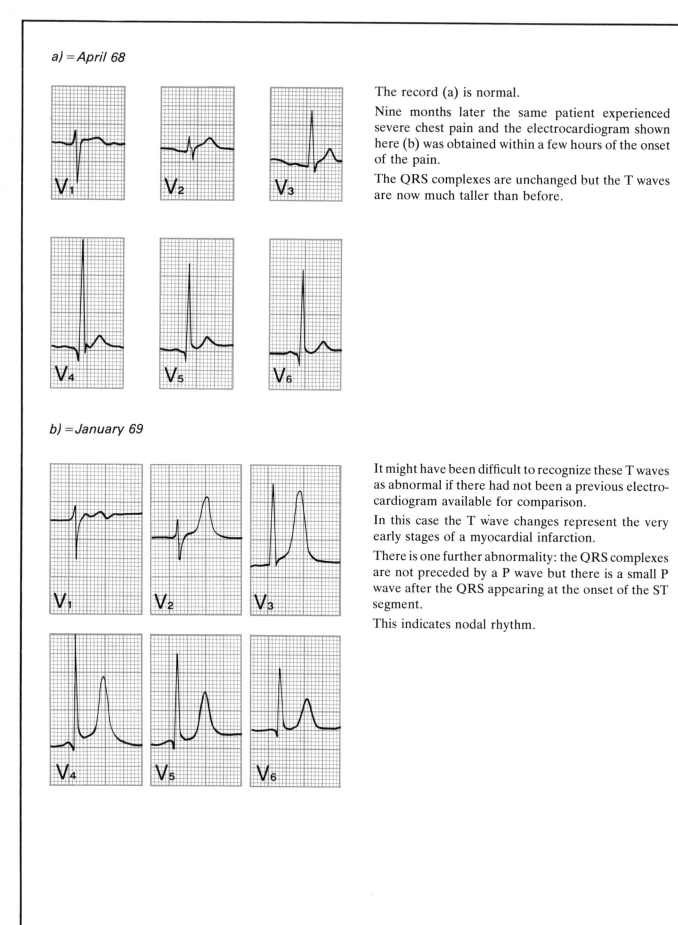

a) = April 68

The record (a) is normal.

Nine months later the same patient experienced severe chest pain and the electrocardiogram shown here (b) was obtained within a few hours of the onset of the pain.

The QRS complexes are unchanged but the T waves are now much taller than before.

b) = January 69

It might have been difficult to recognize these T waves as abnormal if there had not been a previous electrocardiogram available for comparison.

In this case the T wave changes represent the very early stages of a myocardial infarction.

There is one further abnormality: the QRS complexes are not preceded by a P wave but there is a small P wave after the QRS appearing at the onset of the ST segment.

This indicates nodal rhythm.

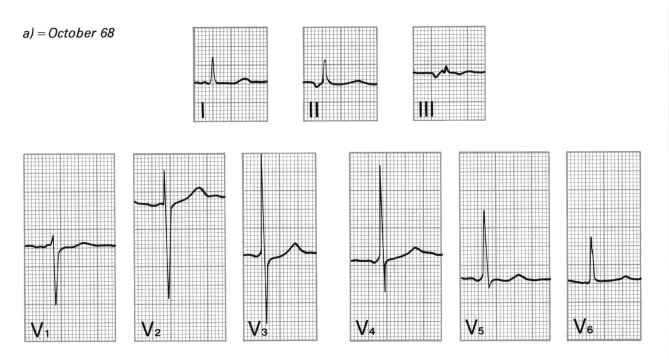

The electrocardiogram (a) shows rather large QRS complexes, the total amplitude of V_3 being 43 mm, and rather small T waves in leads I, V_5 and V_6.

The diagnosis is left ventricular hypertrophy.

The inverted P waves in leads II and III together with the very short PR interval indicate nodal rhythm.

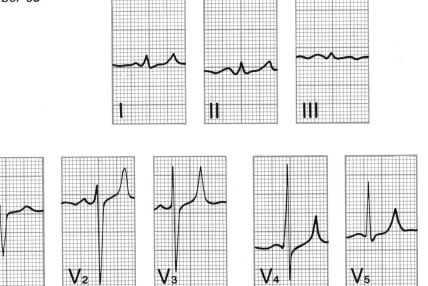

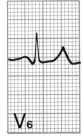

One month later acute renal failure developed and the electrocardiogram (b) now shows tall peaked T waves in many leads.

In this case the abnormal T waves indicate high blood potassium.

Renal dialysis was performed because any further rise in blood potassium might have caused death from ventricular fibrillation.

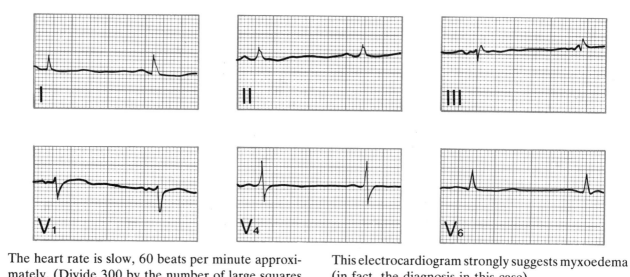

The heart rate is slow, 60 beats per minute approximately. (Divide 300 by the number of large squares between the peaks of two consecutive R waves.)

The QRS complexes are of low voltage throughout and the T waves are of very low amplitude in all leads.

This electrocardiogram strongly suggests myxoedema (in fact, the diagnosis in this case).

Occasionally the electrocardiogram will suggest hypothyroidism when the clinical features are not obvious.

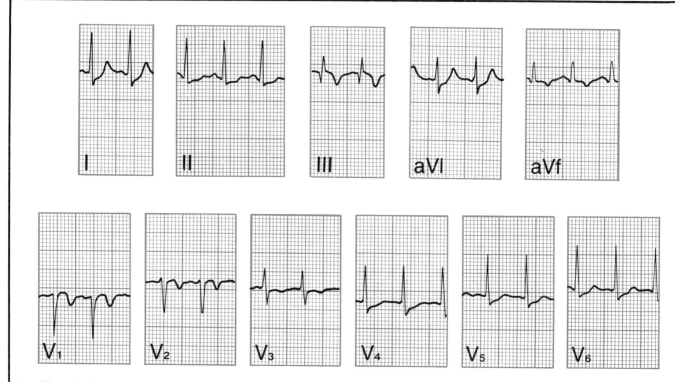

There is T wave inversion in leads III, aVf, V_1, V_2 and V_3. A definite Q is present in lead III, a very small Q in lead aVf and no Q in lead II.

This electrocardiogram, recorded from a man of 45 years of age, could be wrongly diagnosed as indicating an inferior myocardial infarction.

The Q in lead III with T inversion in leads III, aVf and the anterior precordial leads is a typical finding in acute pulmonary embolism which is the diagnosis here.

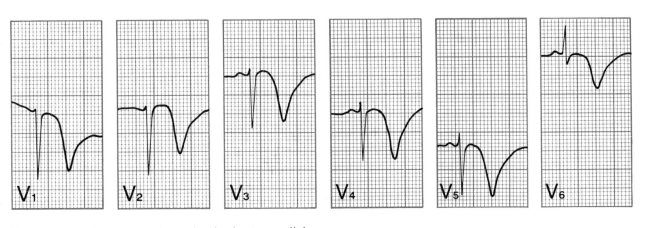

Deep symmetrical T wave inversion in the precordial leads.

The shape of these T waves makes the diagnosis of myocardial infarction probable and this was the diagnosis in this patient.

9. ST and T wave Abnormalities

It is hoped that this description of ST and T abnormalities in left ventricular hypertrophy will serve to amplify and revise much that has been described so far. Further notes have also been added that should be of practical help in the interpretation of the individual electrocardiogram.

Left Ventricular Hypertrophy

Early Changes (Grade 1)

The only abnormality observed is an increase in the voltages of the QRS complexes.

Normal values for the QRS amplitude are exceeded.

The normal values are:

. Sum of R wave in V_5 or V_6 and S wave in V_1 is less than 35 mm.

. R wave in aVf is less than 20 mm.

. Total amplitude of QRS complex in any one lead is less than 35 mm.

More Severe Changes (Grade 2)

The QRS complexes are of abnormally large amplitude and there is depression of the ST segment which is best seen in leads V_5 and V_6 (Figure 9.1).

The T wave remains upright in V_5 but may be rather small. The shape of the ST segment is fairly characteristic, i.e. wave-like, going downwards at first, then upwards.

Note. Subendocardial ischaemia may also cause ST depression, at times indistinguishable from that produced by left ventricular hypertrophy.

The administration of digitalis also produces a very similar effect on the ST segment (Figure 9.2).

These difficulties are resolved as follows:

. The diagnosis of grade 2 left ventricular hypertrophy is made only *in the presence of abnormally large QRS voltages* with ST segment abnormality.

. ST segment depression with normal QRS voltages should be interpreted as myocardial ischaemia.

. Information on the administration of digitalis, digoxin or other related drugs must be obtained.

If the patient has received digitalis within 10 days of record-

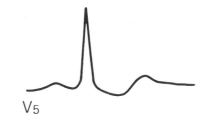

V5

Figure 9.1.

ing the electrocardiogram, the ST segment changes may be due to this drug.

The precise dosage of digitalis administered is not important since the ST sag may appear in the presence of small doses.

This fact is worth remembering, for it explains why it is not possible to judge the adequacy of the digitalis dosage from the electrocardiogram.

At this point the dangers of making a diagnosis from the electrocardiogram without seeing the patient can be illustrated.

Suppose the patient is a very obese man of about 50 years of age with a small, slow-rising arterial pulse and a harsh systolic murmur in the aortic area radiating into the neck, and that the electrocardiogram shows ST segment depression in V_5 with normal amplitude QRS complexes.

The correct interpretation of this electrocardiogram is grade 2 left ventricular hypertrophy, the absence of voltage changes being explained by the patient's obesity.

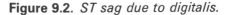

V5

Figure 9.2. *ST sag due to digitalis.*

Fortunately, the general practitioner who records his own electrocardiogram will not be required to report without a full knowledge of his patient but it is well worth remembering that in many of the outpatient ECG schemes the report is given on the electrocardiogram alone.

Finally, if the patient is receiving digitalis and the doctor reporting the electrocardiogram is not aware of this, the dangers of making a completely wrong diagnosis become very great.

Small wonder that the reporter inserts words such as 'the changes suggest', 'the changes are consistent with', etc.

Severe Left Ventricular Hypertrophy (Grade 3)

The QRS complexes are of large amplitude with T wave inversion in V_5, V_6 and usually lead I (Figure 9.3).

Note. The large amplitude of the QRS complexes indicates that the diagnosis is left ventricular hypertrophy.

The T wave changes might otherwise have been interpreted as myocardial ischaemia or infarction.

In ischaemia or infarction the T wave is usually of a different shape, being deeply inverted and symmetrical, but this rule is not absolute.

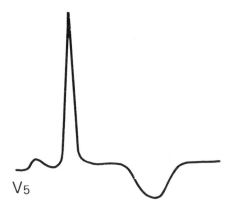

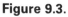

Figure 9.3.

Gross Left Ventricular Hypertrophy (Grade 4)

Left axis deviation and left bundle branch block may, when the clinical features are appropriate, be interpreted as gross left ventricular hypertrophy.

Note. When the QRS complex is grossly disturbed, e.g. in left bundle branch block, an unusual ST and T wave is to be expected (Figure 9.4).

Depolarization of the ventricle is taking an unusual course so repolarization will also take an unusual course.

This is the basis for the terms 'primary' and 'secondary' T wave abnormalities.

Primary T wave abnormality means that the T wave appearances cannot be accounted for purely by the change in the QRS complex.

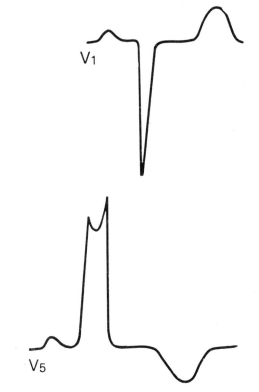

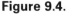

Figure 9.4.

T wave abnormalities are secondary when the abnormal T wave is due to a disturbance of depolarization, i.e. the sole abnormality is in the QRS complex, the T wave change being merely a consequence of this.

In practice, when there is a conduction disturbance in the ventricles, i.e. right or left bundle branch block, it is difficult to differentiate primary from secondary T wave abnormalities. In this case a change in the T wave in successive recordings is often the best guide.

For example, a patient presents with left bundle branch block on the electrocardiogram.

If a second electrocardiogram recorded a few days later shows the same QRS pattern of left bundle branch block but considerable change in the T wave this implies that the T wave appearances were not due to the conduction disturbance. Instead, the diagnosis of recent myocardial ischaemia or infarction would be suggested.

The QT Interval

The QT interval is measured from the beginning of the Q wave to the end of the T wave (Figure 9.5) and occasionally this measurement proves useful in clinical practice.

Unfortunately, there are several difficulties in the measurement and interpretation of the QT interval:

1. The beginning of the Q wave is easily identified but the end of the T wave may be much less distinct. Errors are particularly likely in hypokalaemia. In this condition the T wave is of small amplitude and is followed by a large U

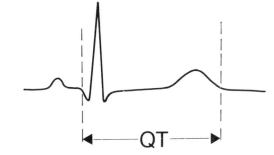

Figure 9.5.

...ave, and it is quite possible to measure the QU interval by ...istake.

The range of normality for the QT interval is wide and ...e interval also varies with cycle length, age and sex. In ...actice, the cycle length (RR interval) and the QT interval ...e measured as precisely as possible from the routine ...ectrocardiogram, and a table which gives the normal ...lue of the QT interval in a patient of that age, sex and ...eart rate is then consulted.

...he QT interval is short in hypercalcaemia and with ...gitalis administration.

...he QT interval is long in hypocalcaemia, hypokalaemia, ...ypothermia, myocarditis, and with quinidine admin-...tration.

Cerebral Disease and the Electrocardiogram

...bnormalities of the ST and T waves are frequently seen in ...sociation with cerebral disease, particularly sub-...rachnoid haemorrhage and intracerebral haemorrhage.

Common findings are ST depression, flat or inverted T waves, marked prolongation of the QT interval and prominent U waves in leads I, V_4, V_5 and V_6.

In these patients careful examination of the heart at autopsy shows no abnormality.

Again, it is important to know the clinical condition of the patient. From the electrocardiogram alone the diagnosis of myocardial ischaemia or infarction might have been made.

Summary

Left ventricular hypertrophy:

Grade 1. Large QRS voltages.

Grade 2. Large QRS voltages with ST depression.

Grade 3. Large QRS voltages with ST depression and T wave inversion.

Grade 4. Left bundle branch block.

Primary T wave abnormalities:

T wave abnormalities due to disease.

Secondary T wave abnormalities:

T wave abnormalities as a natural consequence of alteration in the QRS complex.

QT interval:

1. Prolonged in hypocalcaemia, hypokalaemia, hypothermia, myocarditis and with quinidine administration.

2. Abnormally short in hypercalcaemia and with digitalis administration.

Cerebral disease:

Often causes ST and T wave changes when there is no detectable cardiac abnormality.

Note that in the following examples some of the leads have N/2 written beside them. This indicates that these leads have been recorded at half sensitivity and all measurements of amplitude should be multiplied by two. Thus the R wave in V_5 is 40 mm in height.

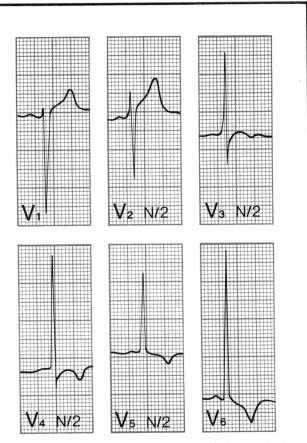

This electrocardiogram shows severe left ventricular hypertrophy (grade 3), with large QRS voltages, ST and T changes.

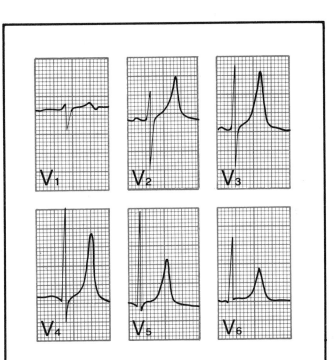

Very tall peaked T waves.

The serum potassium was 8 mEq/l(mmol/l) and the tall T waves are a result of the high serum potassium.

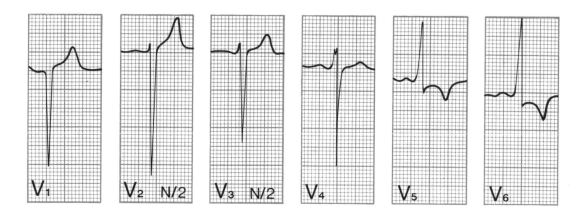

Large amplitude QRS complexes, marked ST and T changes.

There is also some widening of the QRS complexes suggesting an intraventricular conduction defect.

Severe left ventricular hypertrophy (grade 4).

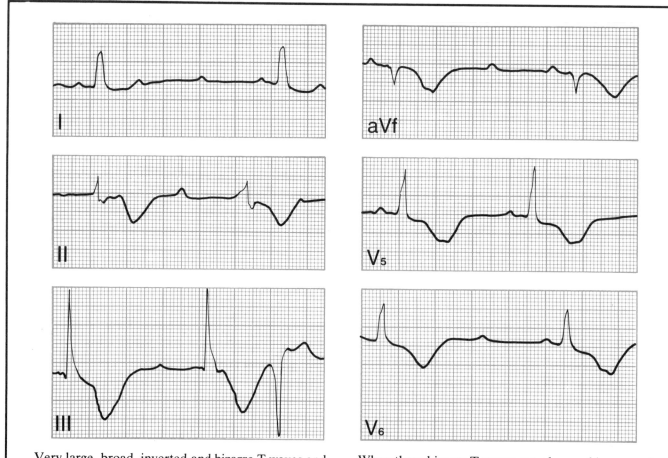

Very large, broad, inverted and bizarre T waves and heart block.

The unusual configuration of the T wave is due partly to a prolongation of the QT interval.

When these bizarre T waves are observed in cases of atrioventricular block they indicate that the patient has had a recent syncopal attack, due either to ventricular standstill or to ventricular fibrillation.

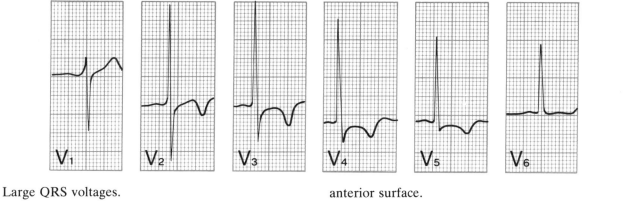

Large QRS voltages.

ST and T changes are unusual, particularly in V_2 and V_3. The deep T wave in V_2 and V_3 becoming less deep in V_4, V_5 and V_6 suggests localized disease in the anterior surface.

The interpretation is left ventricular hypertrophy with the unusual ST and T changes suggesting anterior myocardial infarction or ischaemia.

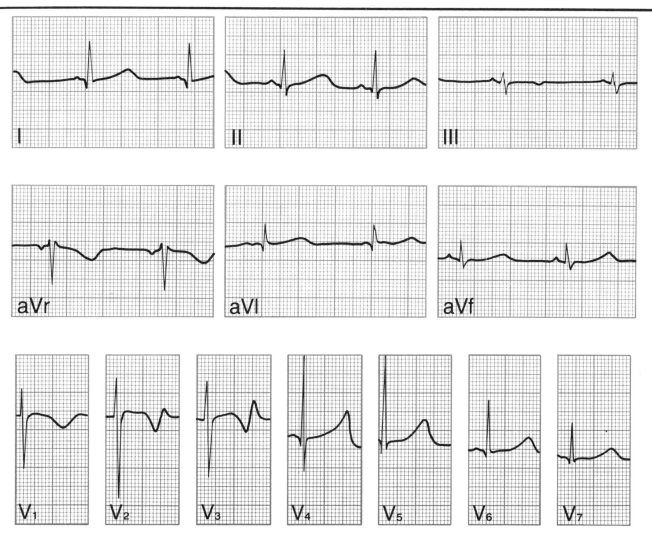

The electrocardiogram of a 10-year-old boy who has a history of attacks of loss of consciousness.

The QT interval is grossly prolonged.

This is an example of a rare inherited condition, often associated with congenital deafness, in which syncopal episodes occur due to transient attacks of ventricular fibrillation. The serum electrolyte levels, including serum calcium, are normal.

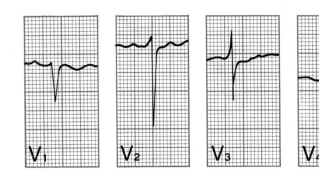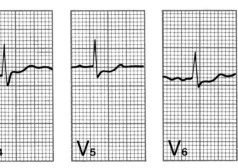

Normal QRS complexes. Straight ST depression of ST segments in leads V₄ and V₅.

The usual interpretation would be subendocardial ischaemia.

This patient, however, was known to have suffered a recent subarachnoid haemorrhage.

In the light of the clinical details the ST changes can be attributed to the subarachnoid haemorrhage. The coronary vessels were in fact normal.

10. Normal and Abnormal Cardiac Rhythms

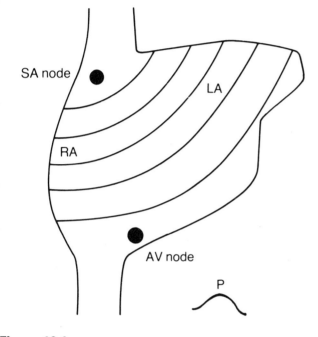

Figure 10.1.

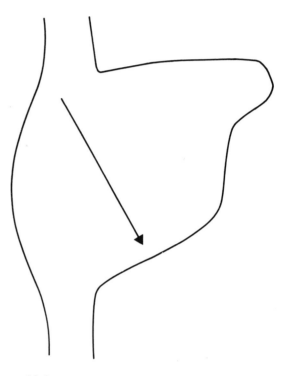

Figure 10.2.

Normal Sinus Rhythm

In normal sinus rhythm the heart rate is controlled by the sinoatrial (SA) node.

The SA node is situated in the right atrium near to the junction of the superior vena cava and the right atrium, and the rate of discharge of the node is under the influence of both sympathetic and parasympathetic nerves. From the SA node the impulse initiating cardiac contraction spreads through the muscle cells of both atria, like a ripple in a pond, to reach the atrioventricular (AV) node.

The AV node lies in the right atrium on the right side of the interatrial septum close to the tricuspid valve.

Figure 10.1 shows the spread of excitation across the atria together with the normal P wave which this excitation wave writes on the electrocardiogram.

In Figure 10.2 the large arrow represents the average direction of spread of this atrial depolarization wave and in Figure 10.3 this arrow has been drawn within the framework of the standard leads.

It should be obvious that this wave of depolarization is travelling towards the left leg and that a large upright deflection will be recorded in lead II.

Lead II is generally the most useful lead for the electrocardiographic diagnosis of normal and abnormal cardiac rhythms because the P wave will be largest and most easily identified in this lead.

However, when the depolarization wave arises in an abnormal site in the atrium and pursues an abnormal direction, lead II may no longer give the best record of atrial depolarization and other leads will be of greater value.

A lead swallowed by the patient so that it lies in the oesophagus close to the atria provides excellent large waves from atrial depolarization. This method was much used in the elucidation of complex arrhythmias but the lead was often rather difficult to position.

When the diagnosis of a complex arrhythmia is required urgently many electrocardiographers now prefer to obtain an electrocardiogram from an electrode placed in the right atrium through an arm vein.

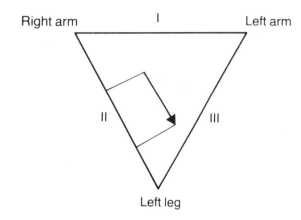

Right arm   I   Left arm

II   III

Left leg

Figure 10.3.

After the arrival of the excitation wave at the AV node it is held up for a brief period. This physiological delay in conduction results in a brief electrically silent period which is represented by a short straight line following the normal P wave on the electrocardiogram (Figure 10.4).

This straight line is isoelectric, is known as the PR segment, and represents the short delay of the impulse in the AV node and in the bundle of His.

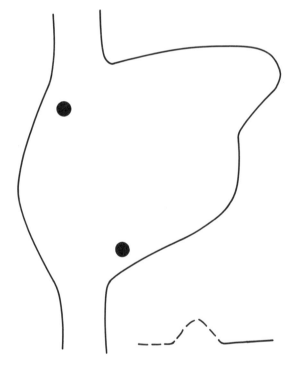

Figure 10.4.

The impulse (Figure 10.5) then leaves the AV node, passes very rapidly down the bundle of His, which divides into two branches (one for each ventricle), and soon reaches the Purkinje fibres through which it directly activates the innermost layers of the myocardium.

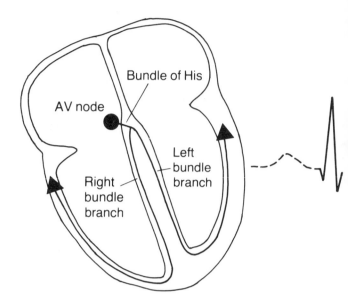

Figure 10.5.

Complete depolarization of the ventricles takes place from the endocardial surface outwards and this ventricular depolarization writes the QRS complex on the electrocardiogram.

Finally, repolarization of the ventricles writes the T wave.

In normal sinus rhythm this sequence of atrial depolarization, followed by ventricular depolarization and repolarization, is repeated indefinitely so that a regular sequence of a P wave, followed by a QRS complex and a T wave, is recorded on the electrocardiogram (Figure 10.6).

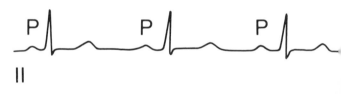

Figure 10.6.

For the electrocardiographic diagnosis of sinus rhythm the following features should be present:

1. A P wave precedes each QRS complex.

2. The PR interval is constant from beat to beat and does not exceed 0.22 seconds in duration.

3. The P wave is upright in lead II.

Sinus Arrhythmia

This is the commonest cause of an irregular pulse and is most marked in the young.

As the patient breathes in the pulse gradually quickens, but it slows again during expiration (Figure 10.7).

The SA node remains in control, initiating impulses at a faster rate during inspiration as a result of sympathetic and

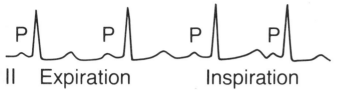

II Expiration   Inspiration

Figure 10.7.

parasympathetic influences.

Each P wave is followed by a QRS complex.

The PR interval is constant and normal.

The P wave is upright in lead II.

Thus all the electrocardiographic features indicating sinus rhythm are fulfilled.

Sinus arrhythmia is a normal finding.

Heart Block

Heart block is present when conduction of the wave of depolarization from the atria to the ventricles is impaired.

Complete interruption of this conduction pathway results in complete heart block.

Lesser degrees of impairment are common and are known as 'latent heart block' (all impulses are conducted but after an excessive delay), and 'partial heart block' (a proportion of impulses are not conducted).

Latent Heart Block (First Degree Heart Block)

The impulse arises in the SA node and spreads over the atria to the AV node in the normal manner.

There is excessive delay in the conduction of the impulse through the AV node and down the bundle of His but every sinoatrial impulse does eventually reach the ventricle and initiates a ventricular contraction.

The ventricles therefore contract regularly at a normal rate.

The electrocardiogram is the best tool for the detection of latent heart block and shows a PR interval greater than 0.22 seconds (5.5 small squares on the electrocardiogram).

Every P wave is followed by a QRS complex.

The P wave is upright in lead II.

The PR interval is constant.

The electrocardiogram therefore shows sinus rhythm (Figure 10.8), but the PR interval is abnormally long and the diagnosis is latent heart block.

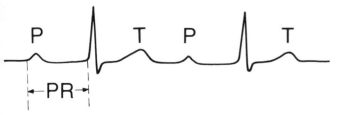

Figure 10.8.

1. Occasionally it can be a normal finding in the presence of a high vagal tone.

2. First degree heart block commonly occurs in acute rheumatic fever where it is an indication of rheumatic carditis.

3. Drugs such as digitalis, beta-blockers and quinidine may produce first degree heart block and the PR interval reverts to normal when the dosage is reduced.

4. Almost any acute infectious disease may cause first degree heart block, e.g. diphtheria which used to be a common cause of heart block.

5. Coronary artery disease and myocardial infarction, particularly inferior myocardial infarction, are common causes of latent heart block.

Significance of Latent Heart Block

The finding of a long PR interval during the course of acute rheumatic fever is an indication of rheumatic carditis. The block nearly always disappears as the disease becomes inactive.

Following myocardial infarction the presence of a long PR interval gives warning of a disturbance of the conducting tissue and this may progress to more severe degrees of heart block, including complete heart block. Fortunately, many patients with first degree heart block after myocardial infarction do not develop complete block.

Any patient who has a long PR interval, however, requires particularly careful supervision. (This is discussed further in Part 11.)

Summary

Standard lead II usually shows the P wave most clearly and, therefore, it is generally the most useful lead for the investigation of a cardiac arrythmia.

The diagnosis of normal sinus rhythm from the electrocardiogram requires that:

1. A P wave must precede each QRS complex.

2. The PR interval is constant and no greater than 0.22 seconds.

3. The P wave is upright in lead II.

Sinus arrhythmia is present when all the criteria for sinus rhythm are fulfilled but the heart rate shows a phasic change, being fast during inspiration and slowing down during expiration. Sinus arrhythmia is a normal finding.

Heart block indicates a disturbance of conduction from the atria to the ventricles. Three stages are recognized:

1. First degree. The PR interval is prolonged.

2. Second degree. Some of the atrial impulses are not conducted to the ventricles.

3. Third degree. Complete interruption of the conduction

pathway between the atria and the ventricles. The atria remain under the influence of the SA node and beat at a normal rate. A subsidiary pacemaker develops in the ventricle and takes over the pacemaking function of the ventricles. Under the control of this subsidiary pacemaker the ventricles beat at a slower rate.

10. Electrocardiograms for Interpretation

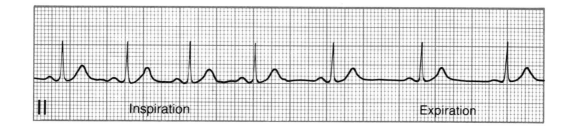

A P wave precedes each QRS complex. The PR interval is 0.16 seconds and is virtually constant. The P wave is upright in lead II.

Sinus rhythm is therefore present.

During inspiration the heart rate is faster than during expiration.

This electrocardiogram shows sinus arrhythmia.

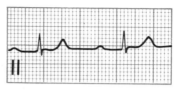

A P wave precedes each QRS complex. The P wave is upright in lead II. The PR interval is constant and this tracing therefore also shows sinus rhythm.

Note, however, that the PR interval is 0.28 seconds. This electrocardiogram shows first degree heart block.

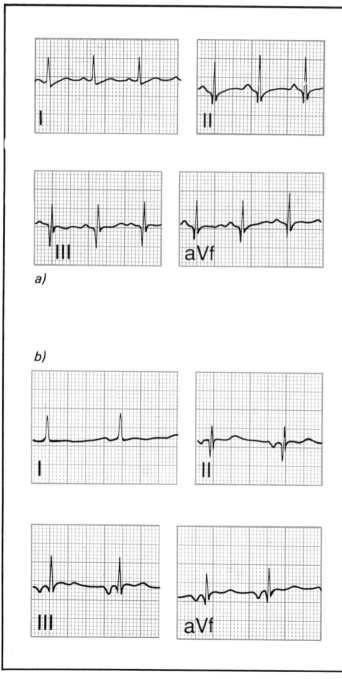

a)

b)

Two electrocardiograms recorded from the same patient are shown.

The electrocardiogram (a) shows normal sinus rhythm and the P waves are upright in leads II, III and aVf.

The electrocardiogram (b) taken one month later shows inverted P waves in leads II, III and aVf.

This indicates that the depolarization wave for the atria is spreading from below upwards, a characteristic feature of nodal rhythm.

Note also that the PR interval is short, 0.12 seconds which is also characteristic for nodal rhythm.

The diagnosis is sinus rhythm in (a) and nodal rhythm in (b).

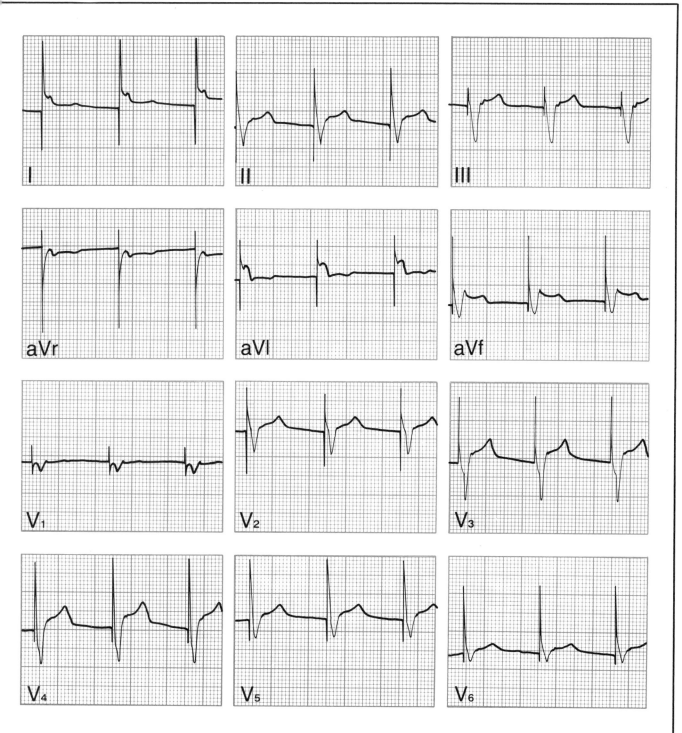

This is the electrocardiogram of a patient in complete heart block who has been treated by the insertion of a permanent cardiac pacemaker.

The sharp deflection preceding each QRS complex is the electrical potential generated by the electronic pacemaker.

The QRS complexes are broad because the impulse passes through the ventricles in a different direction from the normal depolarization wave via the bundle of His and the bundle branches.

11. Heart Block (Atrioventricular Block)

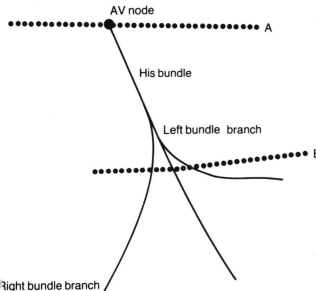

Figure 11.1. *Delay at level A causes type 1 block. Delay at level B causes type 2 block.*

First Degree Heart Block

This was described in Part 10. The prolonged PR interval in first degree heart block is usually caused by a delay in conduction of the atrial impulse through the atrioventricular (AV) node. In the more advanced degrees of heart block the disease may be at the AV node or lower down the conducting system in the His bundle or the bundle branches.

Second Degree Heart Block

In second degree heart block the atria beat at a normal rate under the control of the sinoatrial (SA) node but some of the impulses are completely blocked from the ventricles. The interruption to conduction may be either at the level of the AV node or lower down the conducting system in the bundle of His or the bundle branches (Figure 11.1). As a result of second degree heart block the ventricles beat at a slower rate than the atria. A common type of second degree heart block is 2:1 heart block where the ventricles beat at half the atrial rate. Every alternative P wave fails to be conducted to the ventricles (Figure 11.2).

In 2:1 heart block the electrocardiogram shows alternately

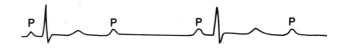

Figure 11.2.

a normal P wave, QRS and T wave, followed by a normal P wave with no QRS or T wave.

The ventricular rate is regular, so the pulse rate is also regular, but slower than normal. If the atrial rate is 80 beats per minute the ventricular rate is 40 beats per minute.

A 3:2 heart block is also encountered clinically, every third atrial depolarization wave being extinguished on its way to the ventricles (Figure 11.3).

The pulse rate is irregular in 3:2 heart block, groups of two beats being separated by a long gap. 3:2 heart block is one cause of bigeminal rhythm (a rhythm in which the pulse beats are grouped in pairs).

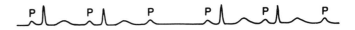

Figure 11.3.

Wenckebach Phenomenon

In second degree heart block the electrocardiogram often indicates the site of the block.

For example, when the AV node is diseased, causing some ventricular beats to be dropped, the Wenckebach phenomenon is observed. This involves a progressive deterioration, beat by beat, in the capacity of the AV node to transmit atrial impulses until one impulse fails to reach the ventricles.

The AV node is able to recover during the time of the blocked impulse and the following impulse is transmitted with little or no delay.

Figure 11.4 shows a progressive lengthening of the PR interval, indicating a progressive deterioration in the conduction time of the AV node.

At X the P wave is not followed by a QRS complex, so a dropped beat results.

After this dropped ventricular beat the P wave is trans-

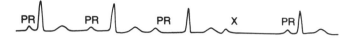

Figure 11.4. *The Wenckebach phenomenon.*

mitted rapidly to the ventricles and has a normal PR interval.

Mobitz Second Degree Heart Block

The Wenckebach type of second degree heart block usually means block in the AV node or high up the bundle of His. Often this type of block is of no great consequence and is associated with acute reversible disease. This type of partial heart block is classified as Mobitz type 1 block to distinguish it from the more serious Mobitz type 2 block.

Mobitz Type 1

The Wenckebach (Mobitz Type 1) partial heart block is seen frequently in myocardial infarction when the infarction involves the inferior surface of the heart (pathological Q waves in leads II, III and aVf).

An infarct in this region is particularly liable to be accompanied by ischaemia of the AV node.

In the great majority of these patients normal conduction is resumed if the acute infarction is survived because the AV node can develop a good alternative blood supply.

Mobitz Type 2

Mobitz Type 2 block is characterized by the constancy of the PR interval in conducted beats. There is no Wenckebach phenomenon.

The site of the block is usually below the bundle of His and this type usually leads to complete heart block with a slow ventricular rate.

Mobitz Type 2 heart block is seen occasionally during the course of an acute anterior myocardial infarction. The area of infarction is always large and involves both bundle branches to cause intermittent heart block. An electrical pacemaker must be inserted at this stage because the condition may well progress to complete heart block and ventricular standstill. The prognosis is poor and 80 per cent of these patients die.

Complete Heart Block

When the abnormality of the conduction system has progressed to complete heart block the atria and the ventricles beat entirely independently.

Atrial rate remains under control of the SA node and accelerates with exertion in the normal manner.

None of the atrial impulses, however, is conducted to the ventricles and the ventricles contract at a slow rate under the control of a subsidiary pacemaker.

The location of the ventricular pacemaker has a considerable influence on the condition of the patient.

When the ventricular pacemaker is high up in the bundle of His the discharge rate is high, usually over 40 beats per minute, the pacemaker is stable and fairly reliable and the QRS complexes are narrow, indicating a normal pathway of conduction down the bundle of His and through the right and left bundle branches to the ventricles.

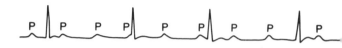

Figure 11.5.

Figure 11.5 shows complete heart block with the ventricular pacemaker high up in the bundle of His.

The QRS complexes are regular but occur at a slower rate than the P waves. The essential feature for the diagnosis of complete heart block is the complete variability of the PR interval.

No constant relationship is to be expected between the P wave and the QRS complex since these are completely independent in complete heart block.

The diagnosis of complete heart block is made from the electrocardiogram when the following features are present:

1. The ventricular rate is slower than the atrial rate.

2. The PR interval is completely random.

In Figure 11.6 the PR interval is completely random and the ventricular rate is slower than the atrial rate.

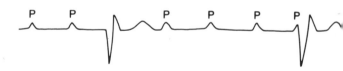

Figure 11.6.

Therefore, there is complete heart block and from the wide bizarre QRS complexes it can be inferred that the pacemaker for the ventricles is located low down in the Purkinje tissue of the ventricles.

This is a serious condition because a low pacemaker drives the ventricles at a rate too slow for the normal everyday activities of the patient and this type of pacemaker is very prone to cease functioning suddenly.

When the pacemaker fails to discharge, ventricular standstill causes abrupt loss of consciousness, succeeded by abrupt return of consciousness when pacemaker activity is resumed (Stokes–Adams attack). Death may occur during one of these attacks, either from prolonged asystole, or from asystole followed by terminal ventricular fibrillation.

Causes of Complete Heart Block

Idiopathic Degeneration

Idiopathic degeneration of the conducting tissues of the heart is the commonest form of complete heart block encountered in the over 60s, and is also encountered occasionally in younger age groups.

The degeneration is confined to the conducting tissue and the myocardium is healthy.

An implanted cardiac pacemaker is required because the idioventricular pacemaker is low down, slow and unreliable. With an implanted pacemaker life expectancy and the quality of life are very good.

Ischaemic Heart Disease

In the first few days following inferior myocardial infarction, second degree heart block of the Mobitz Type 1 variety can progress to complete block.

The ventricular rate is usually adequate, over 40 beats per minute, and sinus rhythm returns spontaneously after the acute phase.

A temporary pacemaker is required only if the patient's general condition deteriorates with the onset of the block.

Much less commonly complete block appears during an acute anterior myocardial infarction, usually preceded by Mobitz Type 2 block. A pacemaker is necessary and despite this the prognosis is usually poor.

Drug Effects

Heart block may be caused by an excess of digitalis, quinidine, propranolol and potassium.

Myocarditis and Some Forms of Cardiomyopathy

Both diphtheria and rheumatic fever during the acute stage have caused transient heart block.

Acute viral infections are suspected as a cause of heart block in occasional cases.

Congenital Complete Heart Block

Heart block is occasionally diagnosed before birth from the low fetal heart rate.

More usually it is picked up at a routine examination of a symptom-free child.

The idioventricular pacemaker is high in the conducting tissues, the ventricular rate is usually over 50 beats per minute and no therapy is required. The ventricular rate may even speed up a little during exercise. Very occasionally an implanted pacemaker is required.

Other Causes

Other causes include trauma to the conducting tissue at cardiac surgery, ankylosing spondylitis and involvement of the bundle of His in calcific aortic stenosis.

Atrioventricular Dissociation

This condition is similar to complete heart block in that the atria and the ventricles beat independently.

The feature differentiating the two types of arrhythmia is the comparison between the atrial and ventricular rates. In atrioventricular dissociation the ventricles are beating at a faster rate than the atria.

The cause of atrioventricular dissociation is an acceleration of the discharge rate from the AV node, which then takes over the pacemaking function for the ventricles.

For this rhythm to appear there must also be a block preventing the retrograde passage of the ventricular depolarization wave into the atria.

In atrioventricular dissociation normal sinus rhythm is usually resumed when the discharge rate of the AV node is slowed.

Summary

First degree (latent heart block):

1. PR interval is prolonged beyond 0.22 seconds (more than 5.5 small squares).

2. Every P wave is followed by a QRS complex.

Second degree heart block (dropped beats):

Some P waves are not followed by a QRS complex.

There are two types of second degree heart block carrying different prognoses:

1. *Mobitz Type 1 (Wenckebach phenomenon)*. The Wenckebach type of second degree heart block is present when each successive P wave is followed by a QRS complex after a progressively lengthening delay until finally one P wave is not transmitted and a ventricular beat is dropped. A reversion to sinus rhythm often occurs.

2. *Mobitz Type 2*. There is no variation in the PR interval in two or more consecutive beats before the dropped beats. This type usually progresses to complete block.

The differentiation between Mobitz Type 1 and Type 2 cannot be made when the rhythm is 2:1 atrioventricular block.

Third degree (complete heart block):

1. No atrial impulses are transmitted to the ventricles.

2. The ventricular rate is slow and regular.

3. The electrocardiogram shows P waves and QRS complexes completely independent of each other.

4. The PR interval is completely variable.

11. Electrocardiograms for Interpretation

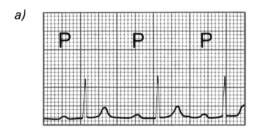

a)

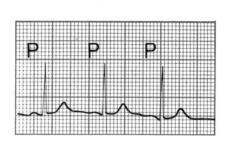

b)

a) Sinus rhythm.

Each P wave is followed by a QRS complex at a constant PR interval. However, the PR interval is 0.28 seconds (seven small squares), which is abnormally long. This electrocardiogram therefore shows first degree heart block.

b) One month later. The PR interval is now 0.16 seconds.

This patient had rheumatic fever with active rheumatic carditis in (a) and the electrocardiogram (b) shows a return to a normal PR interval one month later.

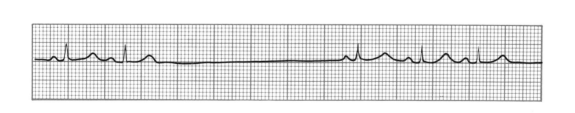

The first two complexes show normal sinus rhythm.

There is then a long period of electrical silence followed by a resumption of sinus rhythm.

The long silent period shows no atrial activity and the diagnosis here is either sinus arrest (the SA node failing to discharge at all during the silent period) or sinoatrial block (the SA node discharging normally but the impulse failing to spread into the atria).

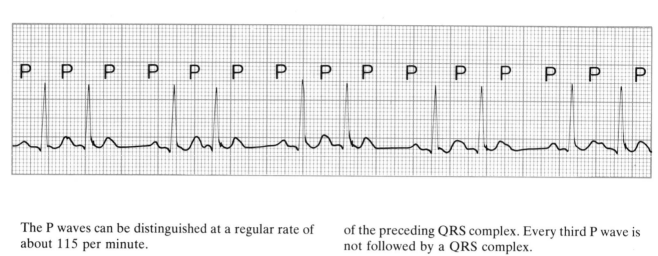

The P waves can be distinguished at a regular rate of about 115 per minute.

Many of the P waves are partly hidden in the T waves of the preceding QRS complex. Every third P wave is not followed by a QRS complex.

This is 3:2 atrioventricular block.

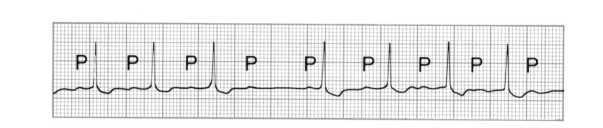

The P waves are small but careful study of the tracing will show that the PR interval gradually lengthens until one P wave is not conducted to the ventricles and is therefore not followed by a QRS complex.

The next P wave is conducted to the ventricles with a fairly short PR interval.

The diagnosis is partial heart block of the Wenckebach type.

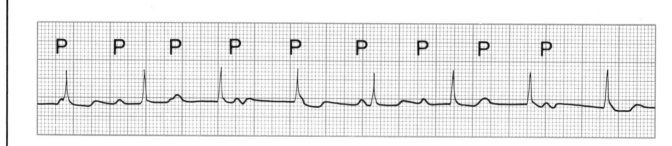

This type of heart block is consistent with normal activities, for the QRS complex is normal and narrow, indicating that the ventricular pacemaker is situated high in the bundle of His, or at the AV node–bundle of His junction.

The P waves are occurring regularly. The QRS complexes also appear regularly but at a rate slower than the P waves. The PR interval is completely variable.

This is complete heart block.

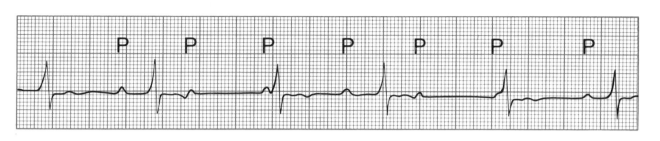

The P waves are regular but the PR interval is completely variable. The QRS complexes, which are abnormally broad, also occur regularly at a rate slower than the P waves.

This is complete heart block with the ventricular pacemaker situated low down in the ventricles. This type of pacemaker is slow and unreliable.

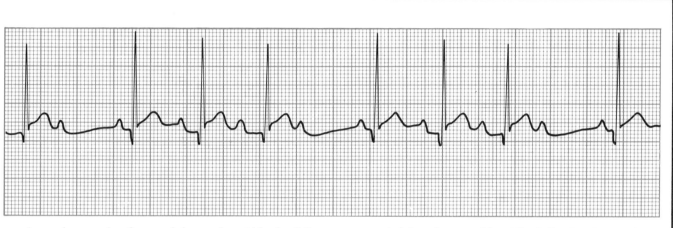

A good example of second degree heart block of the Mobitz Type 1 variety (Wenckebach).

There is progressive lengthening of the PR interval for three cardiac cycles and the fourth P wave is not transmitted to the ventricles. The following P wave is transmitted with a normal PR interval and thereafter there is progressive lengthening of the PR interval.

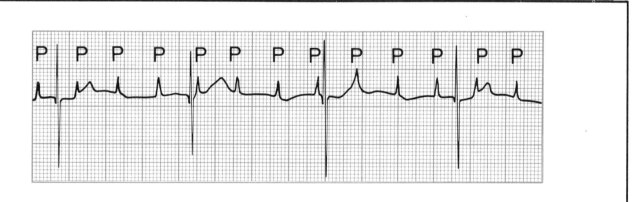

Complete heart block in a four-week-old infant.

The atrial rate is 150 beats per minute, the ventricular rate 42 beats per minute.

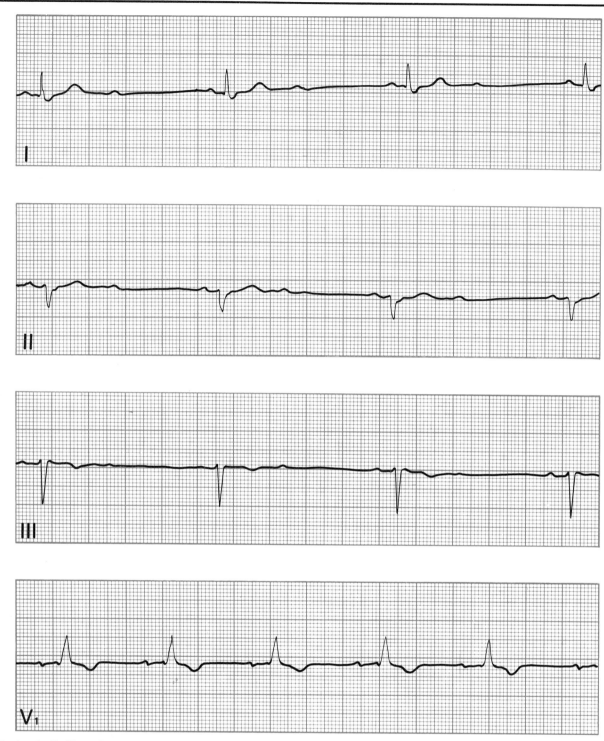

In leads I, II and III there is 2:1 atrioventricular block, with every second P wave failing to reach the ventricles.

In V_1 sinus rhythm has appeared, each P wave stimulating the ventricles after a PR interval of 0.24 seconds. There is a terminal S wave in lead I and a terminal R in V_1, and the QRS complexes are broad: 0.14 seconds in duration. This indicates right bundle branch block.

Finally, the QRS deflection is mainly negative in leads II and III indicating left axis deviation.

Left axis deviation means that the anterior division of the left bundle is blocked. The right bundle is also blocked and, therefore, there is widespread disease of the conducting tissues of the heart.

This patient presented with a history of syncopal attacks due to episodes of complete heart block. Treatment consisted of the implantation of a permanent pacemaker.

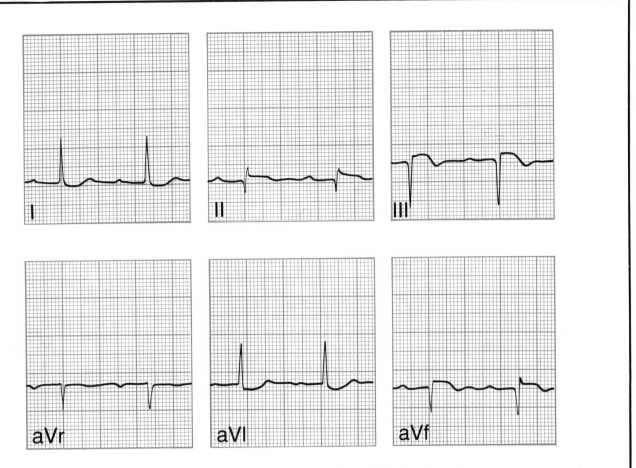

This shows a recent inferior myocardial infarction, with Q waves in leads II, III and aVf. The ST segment is elevated in these leads.

The rhythm is sinus but the PR interval is 0.36 seconds (nine small squares). This first degree heart block is common in acute inferior infarction and does not demand the insertion of a temporary pacemaker.

There is ischaemia of the AV node and the AV node will almost certainly recover over the course of the next few days. The possibility of further deterioration of conduction during the acute stage must be kept in mind but would not necessarily worsen the prognosis.

12. Abnormal Atrial Rhythms

An atrial arrhythmia is present when the impulse initiating cardiac contraction arises somewhere in one or other atrium outside the sinoatrial (SA) node.

An atrial arrhythmia is recognized on the electrocardiogram by the presence of a P wave of abnormal shape followed by a normal QRS complex.

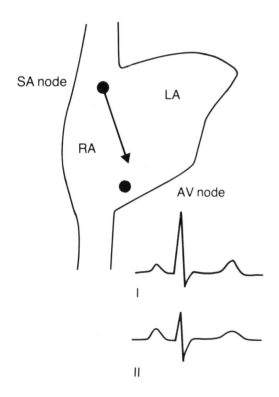

Figure 12.1.

Figure 12.1 is given as a reminder of the normal direction of spread of the wave of depolarization from the SA node over the atria to the atrioventricular (AV) node.

An upright P wave in leads I and II is recorded by the passage of this wave.

Figure 12.2 represents the state of affairs when an irritable focus in the right atrium close to the AV node has taken over.

The SA node is no longer giving out impulses. A focus low down in the right atrium is acting as the pacemaker of the

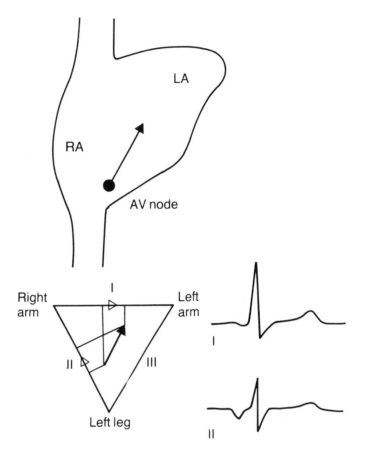

Figure 12.2.

heart and the arrow shows the direction of spread of the depolarization wave over the atria from this new focus. The effect of this new direction of the depolarization wave on leads I and II is also shown in Figure 12.2. The abnormal direction of the spread of the wave has caused the P wave to be inverted in lead II.

The passage of the wave of depolarization through the AV node, the bundle of His and the right and left bundle branches takes place normally. The QRS complexes, therefore, are normal when the arrhythmia arises in the atria.

The diagnosis of an atrial arrhythmia from the electrocardiogram depends upon the recognition of an abnormal configuration of the P wave.

When the ectopic focus acting as pacemaker is situated far

away from the SA node the P wave is obviously abnormal. If the abnormal focus lies near to the SA node only close scrutiny of the P waves, and comparison with the P wave of a tracing taken when the patient was in sinus rhythm, will reveal the abnormality.

Occasional Atrial Extrasystoles

The third heart beat shows an inverted P wave followed by a normal QRS complex (Figure 12.3).

This is an atrial extrasystole. An irritable focus situated low down in the right or left atrium has fired off one impulse and then become dormant again.

The three features of an atrial extrasystole are:

1. The P wave is of abnormal shape.

2. The ectopic impulse arises earlier than the next expected sinus P wave, i.e. it is premature.

3. The compensatory pause after the extrasystole is incomplete.

There is indeed a pause after the extrasystole, before the next sinus P wave is seen, but the sinus beat occurs earlier than would be expected had the heart merely missed one beat altogether.

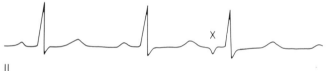

Figure 12.3.

Significance of Atrial Extrasystoles

Occasional atrial extrasystoles are found in the electro-cardiograms of normal hearts and are usually of no significance.

In a patient with chronic rheumatic mitral valve disease the occurrence of frequent atrial extrasystoles may be a warning that atrial fibrillation will soon become established.

Paroxysmal Atrial Tachycardia

In this condition an irritable focus in the atria fires off at a rapid regular rate (usually in the range of 160 to 190 beats per minute).

The focus is outside the SA node and the P wave is therefore of abnormal shape.

Figure 12.4 shows abnormal P waves occurring at a regular fast rate, each P wave being followed by a QRS complex of normal configuration.

The diagnosis of atrial tachycardia presents no difficulty here.

In many patients, however, normal QRS and T complexes occurring at a fast regular rate are seen on the electro-cardiogram, but no P waves may be distinguished. Under these circumstances the diagnosis of atrial tachycardia may be suggested, with abnormal P waves assumed to be present but hidden in the QRS complexes.

Figure 12.4.

Alternatively the irritable focus causing the arrhythmia may be situated in the AV node.

Because of this difficulty in the differentiation of atrial tachycardia from nodal tachycardia, the inclusive term 'supraventricular tachycardia' is often used for either of these two arrhythmias.

As a point of interest, no cells capable of initiating spontaneous depolarization have been found in the AV node but these cells do exist at the junction of the AV node with the bundle of His. The purist has therefore abandoned the term 'nodal tachycardia' in favour of 'junctional tachycardia'.

Significance of Atrial Tachycardia

Commonly atrial tachycardia occurs in the normal heart and does not result in heart failure.

Attacks of paroxysmal tachycardia also occur in heart disease and in these cases heart failure often occurs during the attack.

Urgent treatment may be required when the attacks occur in a diseased heart.

Atrial Flutter

Atrial flutter is produced by an irritable focus in the atria firing impulses at a regular fast rate, usually in the region of 300 impulses per minute.

The AV node and bundle of His do not conduct 300 impulses per minute and usually only every second impulse (2:1 block) or every fourth impulse (4:1 block) reaches the ventricles.

From this description it may appear that atrial flutter is a type of atrial tachycardia at a fast atrial rate. However, since there are many clinical differences between atrial flutter and atrial tachycardia they are regarded as separate conditions.

Atrial flutter is recognized on lead II of the electro-cardiogram.

Lead II shows regular atrial waves at a rate of about 300 per minute with no isoelectric interval between. These regular F (flutter) waves produce a 'picket fence' appearance (Figure 12.5).

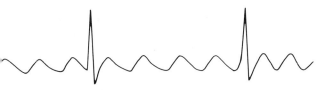

Figure 12.5.

The QRS complexes are normal and occur at a slower rate than the atrial waves.

The ventricular rate is usually 150 beats per minute (2:1 block) or 75 beats per minute (4:1 block) and the ventricles beat regularly unless the degree of block is changing.

The degree of block can be influenced by vagal tone. Carotid sinus massage will often abruptly slow the ventricular rate in this condition.

When the diagnosis is uncertain, a recording of lead II during carotid sinus massage will often slow the ventricular rate and reveal the typical fast F waves which had been obscured by the QRS complexes.

Significance of Atrial Flutter

Atrial flutter usually indicates heart disease. Often the cause is rheumatic mitral valve disease, pulmonary disease, an atrial septal defect or ischaemic heart disease.

Summary

An ectopic atrial focus taking over control of the heart beat for one or more beats is recognized by an abnormal premature P wave followed by a normal QRS complex.

Atrial extrasystole:

1. The P wave is of abnormal shape and occurs early in the cardiac cycle, i.e. earlier than the next expected normal P wave.

2. A normal QRS complex follows the abnormal P wave.

3. There is a short pause, not fully compensatory, before the next normal P wave.

Atrial tachycardia:

1. Abnormal P waves occur at a regular fast rate (160 to 190 per minute).

2. Each P wave is followed by a normal QRS complex.

Nodal tachycardia (junctional tachycardia):

1. Regular QRS complexes occur at a fast rate.

2. No atrial activity is identifiable on the usual leads.

Atrial flutter:

1. Lead II shows regular F waves with no isoelectric interval between them.

2. The QRS complexes are normal and usually appear after every second or fourth F wave.

12. Electrocardiograms for Interpretation

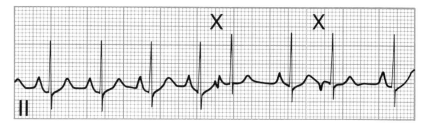

The P wave of the fifth complex (X) is of abnormal shape. This is an atrial extrasystole followed by a normal QRS complex. The pause thereafter is not fully compensatory.

The P wave preceding the seventh complex is again of abnormal shape and is inverted. This is a second atrial extrasystole.

This ECG shows atrial extrasystoles arising from more than one ectopic focus in the atrium.

The P waves are 3 mm in height and triangular, this is a P pulmonale and the diagnosis was cor pulmonale with atrial extrasystoles.

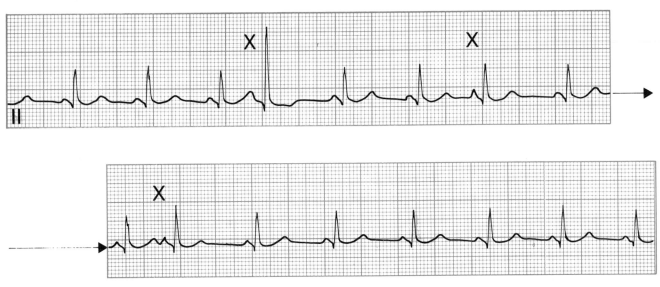

This long record of lead II again shows atrial extrasystoles (marked X).

The first atrial extrasystole is followed by a QRS complex slightly different from the usual. This is because the atrial extrasystole has occurred very early in the cardiac cycle and the ventricular conducting tissue has not had sufficient time to recover from the previous beat.

The impulse from the extrasystole is therefore conducted in an abnormal fashion producing an abnormal QRS complex.

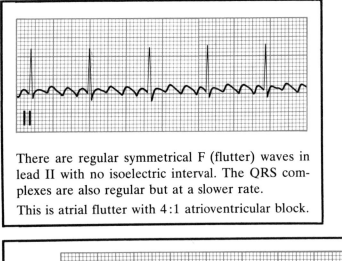

There are regular symmetrical F (flutter) waves in lead II with no isoelectric interval. The QRS complexes are also regular but at a slower rate.

This is atrial flutter with 4:1 atrioventricular block.

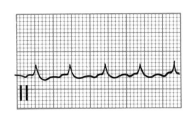

QRS complexes are of normal configuration and occur regularly at a rate of 150 per minute.

Each QRS complex is preceded by a small inverted P wave.

This is an atrial tachycardia.

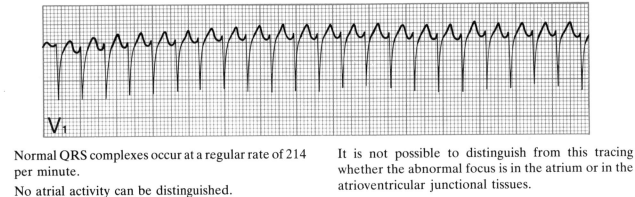

Normal QRS complexes occur at a regular rate of 214 per minute.

No atrial activity can be distinguished.

This is supraventricular tachycardia.

It is not possible to distinguish from this tracing whether the abnormal focus is in the atrium or in the atrioventricular junctional tissues.

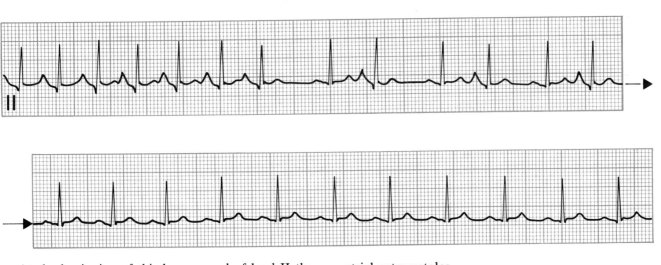

At the beginning of this long record of lead II the QRS complexes are normal and occur regularly at a rate of 136 per minute. The T wave appears sharp and one suspects that there is a P wave fusing with the T wave.

After the eighth complex there is a pause followed by a small P wave and at this point the patient has gone back to sinus rhythm.

The next few seconds show sinus rhythm with coupled atrial extrasystoles.

The bottom strip shows regular normal sinus rhythm.

The T waves during sinus rhythm are of a different configuration from the T waves at the beginning of the recording, confirming that an abnormal P wave was then present.

The diagnosis is paroxysmal atrial tachycardia reverting to sinus rhythm.

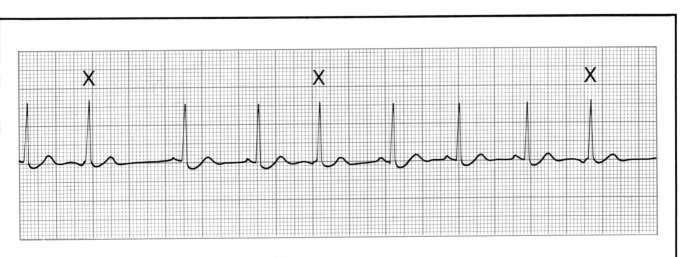

The second, fifth and ninth complexes are atrial extrasystoles.

These all show inverted P waves, which occur early and are followed by a pause which is not fully compensatory.

13. Atrial Fibrillation

In atrial fibrillation the regular wave of depolarization over the atria is abolished and there are no co-ordinated contractions of the atria.

There is a constantly changing pattern of chaotic atrial excitation and the atrioventricular (AV) node is bombarded by stimuli from the fibrillating atria, approximately 500 stimuli per minute.

The AV node is unable to conduct more than 200 stimuli per minute to the ventricles.

In atrial fibrillation the ventricles also beat at a fairly rapid rate, although less than 200 beats per minute.

Many of the stimuli from the atria penetrate the AV node only partially and interfere with the passage of subsequent impulses. This is the reason for the characteristic completely irregular rhythm of the ventricles in atrial fibrillation.

On the electrocardiogram the constantly changing waves of depolarization over the atria produce a continuous, rapidly fluctuating irregular base line.

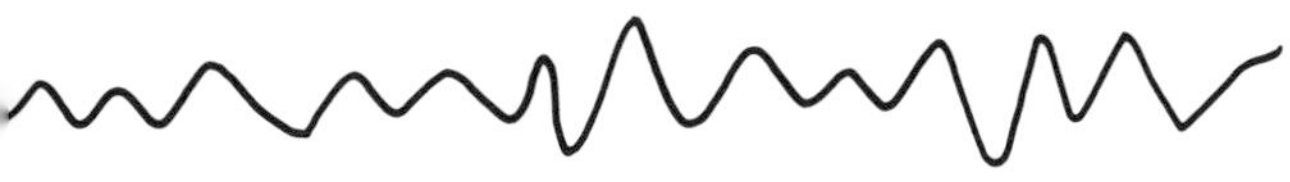

Figure 13.1.

Figure 13.1 is a magnification of the irregular atrial activity which is constantly present in the electrocardiogram from a patient in atrial fibrillation.

The small deflections vary both in rate, size and configuration from moment to moment. They occur at a rate of over 500 per minute and are called 'f' waves. (In Figure 13.1 QRS complexes have been omitted.)

The AV node cannot transmit all the atrial impulses, but any impulse that is conducted reaches the ventricles through the normal pathway, i.e. down the bundle of His, through the right and left bundle branches to the Purkinje fibres and thence to the ventricular myocardium.

The spread of the depolarization wave through the ventricles is therefore normal resulting in normal QRS and T complexes on the electrocardiogram.

Atrial fibrillation is diagnosed from the electrocardiogram by two criteria:

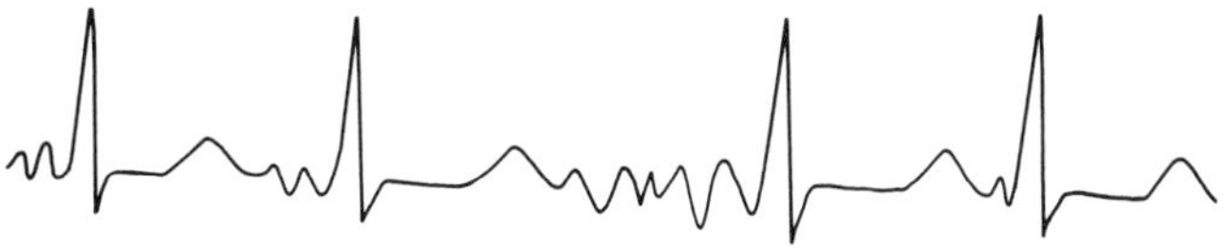

Figure 13.2.

1. The base line shows fast irregular undulations.

2. The QRS and T complexes are of normal configuration but there is a complete irregularity in the rate of the ventricular beats, shown as a random variation in the distances between the QRS complexes (see Figure 13.2).

Note. Occasionally the electrocardiogram recorded from a patient with parkinsonism will cause diagnostic difficulty. The somatic muscular tremor of this condition gives rise to an undulating base line on the electrocardiogram which may easily be mistaken for atrial fibrillation. The QRS complexes occur regularly, however, and a P wave may be distinguished from time to time above the muscle tremor. Finally, the doctor who records his own electrocardiogram will be well aware that his patient has a tremor.

Flutter-fibrillation

Occasionally, in atrial fibrillation, the fibrillary waves on the electrocardiogram become coarse and rhythmic enough to resemble atrial flutter for brief periods. Some observers call this 'impure flutter' or 'flutter-fibrillation'.

However, simultaneous electrocardiographic leads often show that while flutter-like waves are being written in one lead typical fibrillation waves are seen in another.

It is best to reserve the term flutter for the typical case and call the impure examples 'atrial fibrillation'.

Causes of Atrial Fibrillation

Two factors favour the establishment of atrial fibrillation:

1. Enlargement of the left or right atrium, which allows circus movement to become established.

2. Disease causing fibrosis of the atrial myocardium and favouring the fragmentation of its electrical activity.

One or both of these factors is present in the common causes of atrial fibrillation which include rheumatic heart disease, particularly when the mitral valve is affected, hypertensive and ischaemic heart disease, and thyrotoxic heart disease.

Treatment of Atrial Fibrillation

The rapid irregular ventricular rate reduces cardiac efficiency and the usual therapy is to give digoxin which reduces the capacity of the AV node to conduct atrial stimuli to the ventricles. The dosage of digoxin is increased until the ventricular rate is about 80 beats per minute.

In some patients it is worth while to restore sinus rhythm by giving a direct current shock, but atrial fibrillation will soon recur unless the patient has been carefully selected. Usually only patients in whom the cause of the atrial fibrillation has been removed, e.g. after cure of thyrotoxicosis or after a successful mitral valvotomy in a young patient, are suitable.

Use of Synchronized Direct Current Shock in Atrial Fibrillation

A large direct current shock is applied across the chest of the anaesthetized patient and this immediately depolarizes all the atrial cells and abolishes all circus movements.

The next normal discharge from the sinoatrial (SA) node re-establishes sinus rhythm.

An 85 per cent success rate in restoring sinus rhythm has been obtained using this treatment, but atrial fibrillation will soon recur unless the patient has been carefully selected.

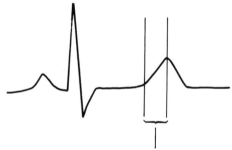

Vulnerable period

Figure 13.3.

The ascending limb of the T wave is known as the vulnerable period of the heart (Figure 13.3).

It is important that the direct current shock should not be given during this vulnerable period, because there is a danger of ventricular fibrillation if a stimulus is administered during the ascending limb of the T wave.

A synchronized shock is therefore given, automatically fired by the R wave of the patient's electrocardiogram, thereby giving the shock well away from the T wave (Figure 13.4).

Serious cardiac arrhythmias can result from the admin-

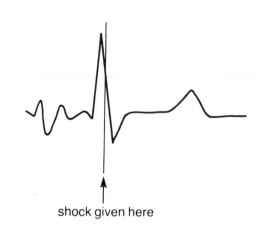

shock given here

Figure 13.4.

istration of a direct current shock in the presence of digitalis toxicity.

Digitalis and the Electrocardiogram

Whenever the patient is receiving digitalis there is a sagging depression of the ST segment with reduction in amplitude of the T wave (Figure 13.5).

The degree of ST depression bears little or no relation to the degree of digitalization. This effect on the electrocardiogram cannot be used to judge the dosage of digitalis.

The electrocardiogram may, however, be of great value in showing arrhythmias due to digitalis toxicity, and on occasions the electrocardiogram may give the first clear evidence of digitalis toxicity.

An excess of digitalis can produce any arrhythmia, including atrial fibrillation and complete heart block. The following arrhythmias are often a manifestation of digitalis toxicity.

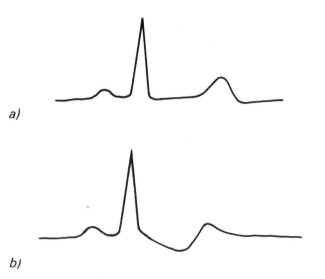

a)

b)

Figure 13.5. a) Before and b) after digitalis therapy. Digitalis causes a downward sag of the ST segment and reduction in height of the T wave.

104

Coupled Ventricular Extrasystoles

ery second QRS complex is wide and bizarre (Figure
.6), indicating that the focus initiating the impulse lies
mewhere in the ventricles.

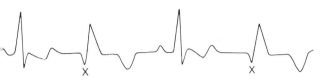

gure 13.6.

Paroxysmal Atrial Tachycardia with Block

his arrhythmia frequently resembles atrial flutter and may
 indistinguishable from it (Figure 13.7).

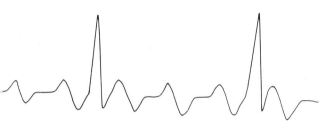

igure 13.7.

sually in paroxysmal atrial tachycardia with block the
ctopic focus in the atria fires off at a rather slower rate than
 atrial flutter, so that lead II of the electrocardiogram
ows atrial waves at a rate of approximately 200 per
inute.

he atrial rate may vary a little—a most unusual finding in
ue flutter—and ventricular extrasystoles often occur.

here is usually an isoelectric line between the atrial waves
in lead II in atrial tachycardia with block whereas in atrial
flutter the base line continually undulates.

When paroxysmal atrial tachycardia with block is seen on
the electrocardiogram the digitalis therapy must be stopped
immediately.

Summary

Atrial fibrillation:

1. The regular wave of depolarization over the atria is
abolished.

2. The AV node cannot transmit all the atrial impulses.

3. The ventricular rhythm is irregular.

Atrial fibrillation is recognized by:

1. Fast irregular undulation of the base line.

2. Random variation in the distance between QRS complexes.

Factors leading to atrial fibrillation:

1. Enlargement of the left or right atrium.

2. Fibrosis of the atrial myocardium due to disease.

Treatment of atrial fibrillation:

1. Digoxin administration to reduce AV node conduction
capacity.

2. DC shock to restore sinus rhythm.

Flutter-fibrillation:

Coarse, rhythmic fibrillary waves resembling atrial flutter.

Digitalis effects:

The following arrhythmias may occur as a manifestation of
digitalis toxicity.

1. *Coupled ventricular extrasystoles*. Every second QRS
complex is wide and bizarre.

2. *Paroxysmal atrial tachycardia with block*. Resembles
atrial flutter. In lead II atrial waves occur at a rate of about
200 per minute.

13. Electrocardiograms for Interpretation

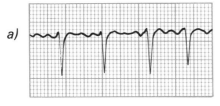 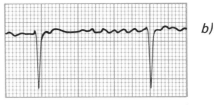

a)

b)

Atrial fibrillation.

The base line shows fast irregular undulation from the fibrillating atria.

In (a) the ventricular rate is fast and irregular.

In (b), which is recorded from the same patient after digitalis has been given, the fast irregular base line fluctuation persists, indicating atrial fibrillation as before but the ventricular rate has been slowed.

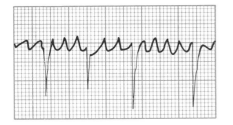

The ventricular complexes occur irregularly.

The base line shows fast waves which vary both in size and rate.

The diagnosis atrial fibrillation is preferred to the term 'flutter-fibrillation'.

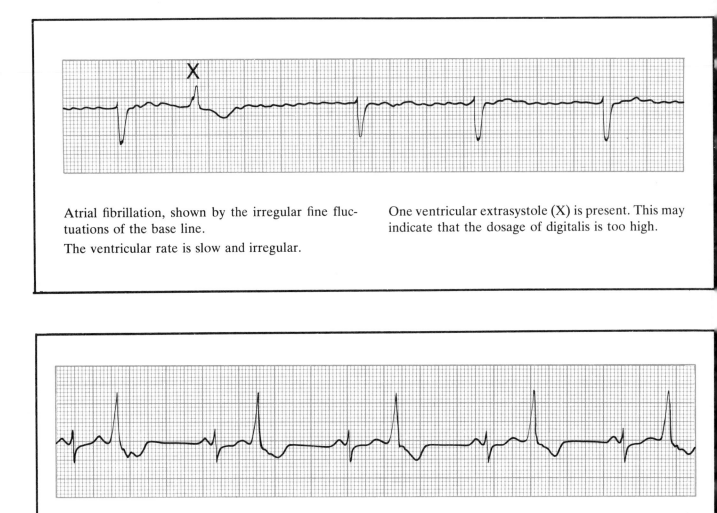

Atrial fibrillation, shown by the irregular fine fluctuations of the base line.

The ventricular rate is slow and irregular.

One ventricular extrasystole (X) is present. This may indicate that the dosage of digitalis is too high.

Sinus rhythm, but every second beat is wide and bizarre and is followed by a compensatory pause.

This is coupled ventricular extrasystoles and indicates that the dosage of digitalis is excessive.

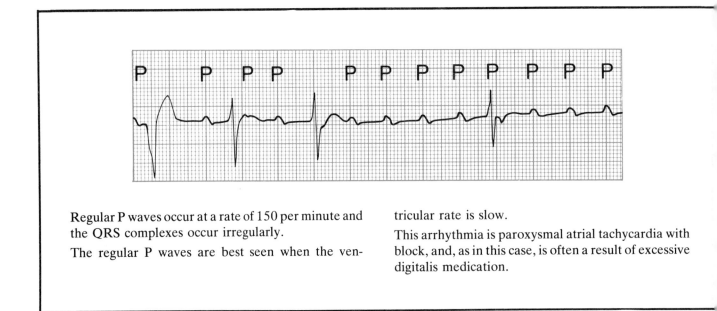

Regular P waves occur at a rate of 150 per minute and the QRS complexes occur irregularly.

The regular P waves are best seen when the ventricular rate is slow.

This arrhythmia is paroxysmal atrial tachycardia with block, and, as in this case, is often a result of excessive digitalis medication.

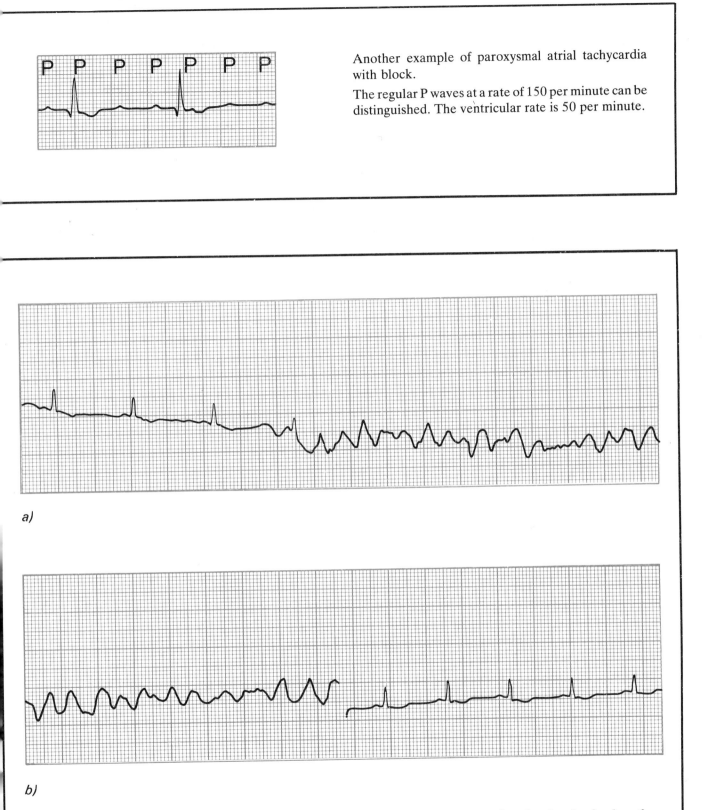

Another example of paroxysmal atrial tachycardia with block.

The regular P waves at a rate of 150 per minute can be distinguished. The ventricular rate is 50 per minute.

a)

b)

The tracing (a) shows the sudden onset of ventricular fibrillation in a patient previously in sinus rhythm.

A direct current shock was administered immediately (b), and this restored sinus rhythm.

There is no need to synchronize the shock when the rhythm is ventricular fibrillation nor is general anaesthesia necessary because the patient rapidly becomes unconscious with the onset of this rhythm.

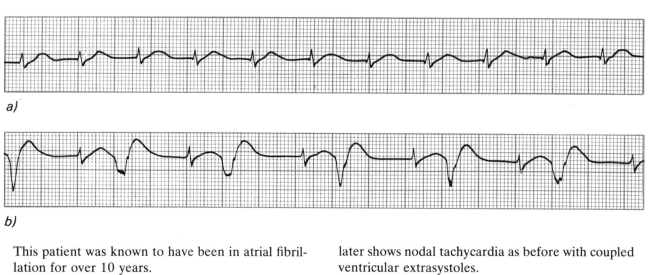

a)

b)

This patient was known to have been in atrial fibrillation for over 10 years.

On admission to hospital the pulse rate was regular and the electrocardiogram (a) shows a nodal tachycardia at a rate of 80 per minute.

An electrocardiogram (b) obtained some minutes later shows nodal tachycardia as before with coupled ventricular extrasystoles.

The dosage of digitalis had been slightly too high and over the course of months had built up to a toxic level. After five days without digitalis this patient reverted to her usual rhythm, atrial fibrillation.

14. Ventricular Arrhythmias

Ventricular Extrasystoles (Ventricular Premature Beats)

When an irritable focus in any part of the ventricular myocardium activates the ventricles before the arrival of the next normal wave of depolarization from the atria a ventricular extrasystole is produced (Figure 14.1).

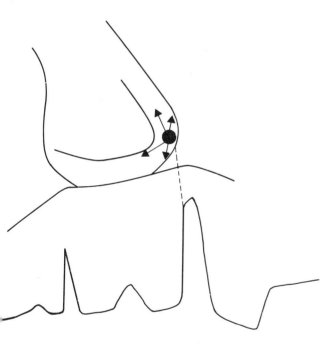

Figure 14.1. *The second QRS is broad and abnormal in shape and is the result of one impulse spreading from an ectopic focus in the ventricle.*

Since the ventricles are activated prematurely the electrocardiogram reveals a QRS complex occurring sooner than expected in the cardiac cycle.

Furthermore, this early QRS complex is of a wide and abnormal shape. The wave of depolarization of the ventricles arises in the irritable focus within the right or left ventricle and pursues a slow abnormal course through the myocardium of both ventricles.

Usually this wave of depolarization in the ventricles does not conduct upwards to the atria, so the atrial rate, and the atrial P waves, are not affected.

On the electrocardiogram a ventricular extrasystole has the following characteristics:

1. A broad QRS complex of unusual shape appears sooner than the next expected QRS complex and is not preceded by a P wave.

2. There is a long pause after the abnormal QRS complex before normal beating is resumed. In electrocardiographic terms, the pause is 'fully compensatory'.

The explanation of the long pause is simply that the next normal wave of depolarization from the atria arrives at the ventricles at a time when they are unable to respond because they are refractory to all stimuli during and immediately after the ventricular extrasystole. Normal rhythm is resumed only with the second atrial wave following the extrasystole.

On the electrocardiogram the distance between the sinus beats preceding and following the ventricular extrasystole is exactly twice the regular distance (Figure 14.2). This is the 'fully compensatory' pause.

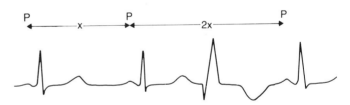

Figure 14.2.

Ventricular extrasystoles are common in association with any form of organic heart disease and may also be produced by digitalis intoxication.

Occasionally ventricular extrasystoles occur in a normal heart.

Frequent ventricular extrasystoles are the rule immediately following myocardial infarction and may require treatment to prevent the appearance of ventricular tachycardia and ventricular fibrillation. Figure 14.3 shows a particularly dangerous type of extrasystole.

Ventricular Tachycardia

Ventricular tachycardia indicates serious heart disease.

The cause of ventricular tachycardia may be either an irrit-

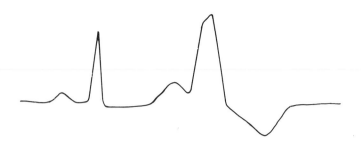

Figure 14.3 *A ventricular extrasystole occurring on the T wave of the previous beat. This is the 'R on T' phenomenon, and after myocardial infarction may precipitate ventricular tachycardia or ventricular fibrillation.*

able focus in the ventricle discharging regularly at a fast rate or a re-entry effect, whereby a pathway in the ventricles allows an impulse to circulate indefinitely.

The ventricular rate may be very fast, over 200 beats per minute, quite slow in the region of 100 beats per minute, or any rate between these two extremes.

Classically the atria remain under control of the sinoatrial (SA) node and there is a block to retrograde conduction of ventricular impulses to the atria.

Thus the ventricles beat at a fast regular rate while the atria beat at a rate of 70 to 80 beats per minute.

It must be admitted that in many cases retrograde conduction to the atria does take place and the atria then follow the ventricles at the same rate.

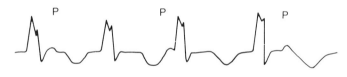

Figure 14.4.

The classical appearances of ventricular tachycardia (Figure 14.4) are:

1. The QRS complexes occur at a fast, regular rate. Each QRS complex is identical in configuration but, since the ventricles are being depolarized in an abnormal fashion, the QRS complexes are broad and bizarre in appearance.

2. Careful scrutiny of the tracing should reveal small P waves occurring at a slower, regular rate and appearing as small deflections at various points on the QRS complexes.

Often it is not possible to distinguish P waves in any of the 12 standard leads of the electrocardiogram, because the P waves are small and are obliterated by the large, fast deflections of the QRS complexes.

Atrial activity may then be defined by recording a lead from the oesophagus at the level of the atria, or, alternatively, an electrode may be placed in the right atrium from an arm

vein and this will also provide a large signal from atr depolarization.

At this point the reader may well ask why the demo stration of atrioventricular dissociation is helpful in t diagnosis of ventricular tachycardia.

The differential diagnosis between supraventricular a ventricular tachycardia would appear to be simple.

In supraventricular tachycardia the impulse enters the ve tricles through the bundle of His and spreads by norm pathways through the ventricular myocardium. The QF complexes are therefore normal in configuration.

Conversely, in ventricular tachycardia the ventricles a depolarized by abnormal pathways, the impulse arisir somewhere in the ventricular myocardium, and the QF complexes are wide and bizarre.

Unfortunately this simple differentiating feature is mo unreliable.

In many patients with a supraventricular tachycardia, functional bundle branch block develops, usually in th right bundle.

The affected bundle is unable to conduct the fast stream impulses from the atria into the ventricle with the resu that the QRS complexes become wide due to function bundle branch block.

These wide QRS complexes mimic ventricular tachycardia

It is this feature of aberrant ventricular conduction tha makes the differentiation of supraventricular from ve tricular arrhythmias so very difficult and at times almo impossible.

Features suggesting that the diagnosis is ventricular tachy cardia include:

1. The demonstration of P waves at a slower rate. Thes can be seen in over 20 per cent of cases of ventricula tachycardia.

2. The finding, before or after the tachycardia, of ver tricular extrasystoles which have the same appearance a the abnormal QRS complexes during the paroxysm.

3. The occurrence of fusion beats during the tachycardi A fusion beat occurs when a sinoatrial beat enters th ventricle at about the same time as the ventricle is stimu lated by the ventricular focus. A QRS complex which par tially resembles both a normal sinus beat and the QR during the tachycardia results.

In very difficult cases, particularly when there are recurren attacks, His bundle studies will help.

The His Bundle Electrogram

An electrode catheter is passed up the femoral vein unti the tip is in the right ventricle, lying against the bundle o His.

Three distinct episodes of electrical activity are recorde (Figure 14.5). A is the atrial deflection, H is the impuls from the bundle of His, and QRS is the electrical activit om the ventricles. It is now possible to measure the time interval AH which represents the time for conduction from the onset of atrial depolarization until the impulse reaches the bundle of His, and includes atrial depolarization time and atrioventricular (AV) node conduction time.

The interval HV is the conduction time from the bundle of His through the bundle branches to the onset of depolarization of the ventricular myocardium.

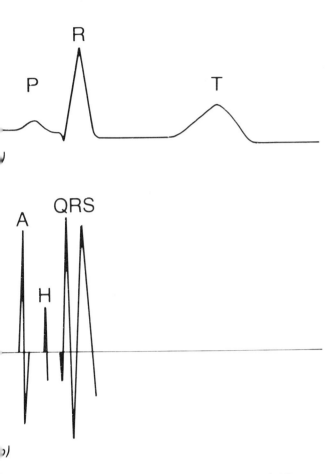

Figure 14.5. a) Electrocardiogram tracing, b) His bundle electrogram.

Using this technique it is possible to demonstrate the site of any heart block and to differentiate between supraventricular and ventricular tachycardia.

When the QRS complex is preceded by a His bundle spike with a near normal HQ interval the tachycardia is supraventricular.

Idioventricular Tachycardia

This is a common finding during acute myocardial infarction and does not usually require specific therapy.

An ectopic ventricular focus discharges at a rate slightly above the prevailing sinus rate causing short periods of broad QRS complexes which are dissociated from the P waves but which occur at a rate of under 100 beats per minute.

Ventricular Fibrillation

Depolarization of the ventricles becomes irregular and fragmented and there is no co-ordinated heart beat.

The rapid sporadic depolarization of isolated parts of the ventricles produces rapid irregular and bizarre complexes of the electrocardiogram (Figure 14.6).

Ventricular fibrillation is a common cause of sudden death in acute myocardial infarction and also occurs terminally in many types of organic heart disease.

Occasionally digitalis, quinidine, electrolyte abnormalities, hypothermia or electrocution are the cause of ventricular fibrillation.

It is important to recognize the pattern produced by ventricular fibrillation on the electrocardiogram because in all cases of sudden cardiac arrest an electrocardiogram should be used to distinguish between ventricular fibrillation and ventricular standstill.

Figure 14.6.

The Wolff–Parkinson–White Syndrome

The Wolff–Parkinson–White syndrome is an electrocardiographic abnormality which is seen only occasionally and usually in people who have normal hearts and a normal life expectancy.

However, it is important that this syndrome be recognized for two reasons:

1. There is an abnormal initial deflection of the QRS complex which may be mistaken for pathological Q waves. Therefore, the patient may be wrongly diagnosed as having a myocardial infarct.

2. Patients with this syndrome are prone to attacks of supraventricular tachycardia which respond to vagal stimulation but not to digitalis.

The Wolff–Parkinson–White syndrome has the following characteristics:

1. The rhythm is sinus and the PR interval is short, less than 0.12 seconds (three small squares on the electrocardiogram).

2. The initial part of the QRS complex is slurred and is called the delta wave (Figure 14.7)

3. Patients with the Wolff–Parkinson–White syndrome are

113

Figure 14.7.

prone to attacks of supraventricular tachycardia.

Patients with this syndrome have an accessory pathway of specialized conduction tissue which bypasses the AV node and connects the atria directly to the ventricles (Figure 14.8)

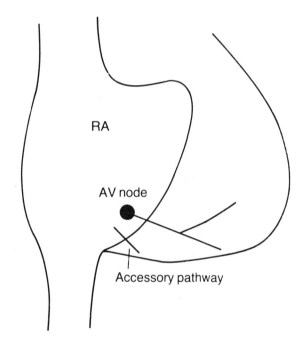

Figure 14.8.

The impulse from the atria undergoes the usual period of delay in the AV node before being passed down the bundle of His to the ventricles. However, during this latent period the wave of depolarization is transmitted down the accessory pathway to activate the ventricle in that region.

Early ventricular depolarization in the region of the accessory pathway produces a slurred initial deflection on the QRS, the delta wave, and this wave merges with the normal QRS complex written by the depolarization of the ventricles which is taking place by normal pathways.

Summary

A ventricular extrasystole, also called a ventricular premature beat, has the following characteristics:

1. The QRS complex is broad and occurs early.

2. There is no P wave before the broad complex and the long pause after the extrasystole is fully compensatory.

Ventricular tachycardia:

1. Seen on the electrocardiogram as a succession of QRS complexes occurring regularly at a rapid rate (usually over 100 per minute).

2. The QRS complexes are wide and of unusual appearance.

3. Careful scrutiny of the tracing may reveal regular P waves occurring at a slower rate which appear as small deflections at various points on the QRS complexes.

4. Broad QRS complexes alone are not sufficient for the diagnosis of ventricular tachycardia.

Supraventricular tachycardia:

Frequently complicated by a functional bundle branch block in the ventricles which produces wide QRS complexes resembling ventricular tachycardia.

His bundle electrogram studies may help to differentiate between ventricular and supraventricular tachycardia.

Ventricular fibrillation:

Produces irregular, rapid and bizarre deflections on the electrocardiogram.

The Wolff–Parkinson–White syndrome is characterized by:

1. A short PR interval.

2. A slurred initial deflection of the QRS complex called the delta wave.

3. A tendency to attacks of supraventricular tachycardia.

14. Electrocardiograms for Interpretation

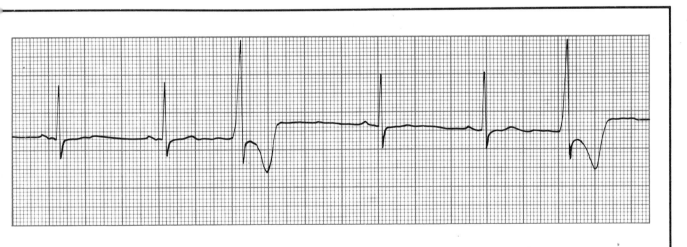

The third and sixth QRS complexes are large, broad and premature, occurring earlier than the next expected sinus beat.

The pause after the premature beat is long and is fully compensatory.

This tracing shows two ventricular extrasystoles. They are identical in appearance and therefore arise from the same ventricular focus.

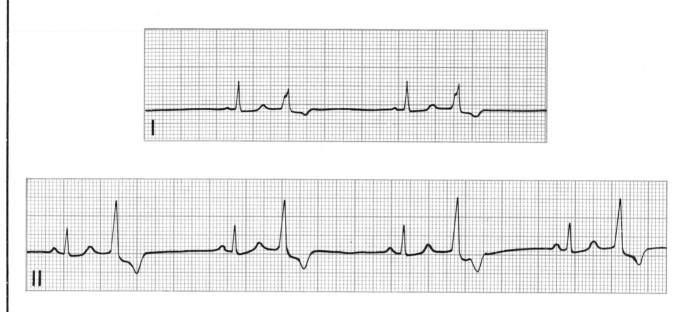

This electrocardiogram shows coupled ventricular extrasystoles.

In lead I the first beat is clearly sinus in origin as there is a normal P wave followed by a normal narrow QRS complex.

The next QRS complex is broad and of abnormal shape. This QRS complex, which is not preceded by a P wave, is a ventricular extrasystole.

The next beat is sinus and the next again is another ventricular extrasystole.

In lead II the pattern of sinus beat alternating with ventricular extrasystole is again seen.

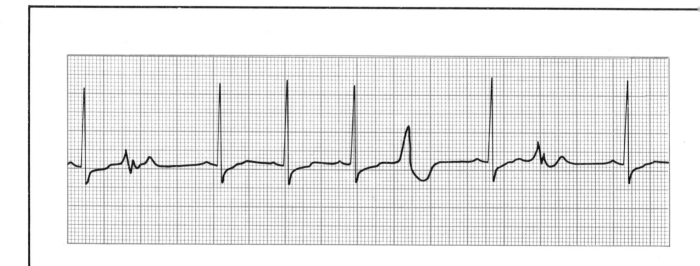

The second, sixth and eighth QRS complexes are broad and of a bizarre shape. Each occurs prematurely and there is a fully compensatory pause after the extrasystole.

These are ventricular extrasystoles and since their shapes are so different they must arise from more than one focus in the ventricles.

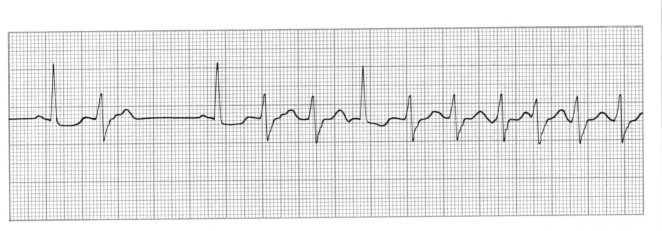

The second QRS complex is a ventricular extrasystole occurring close to the T wave of the preceding sinus beat.

The fourth QRS complex is an extrasystole on the T wave of the preceding beat and this triggers off ventricular tachycardia.

Note that the shape of the QRS complexes during the ventricular tachycardia is practically identical to the QRS of the ventricular extrasystole. The one narrow, normal-looking complex during the ventricular tachycardia is a capture beat—a sinus impulse which has reached the ventricles at a time when the ventricle was not refractory.

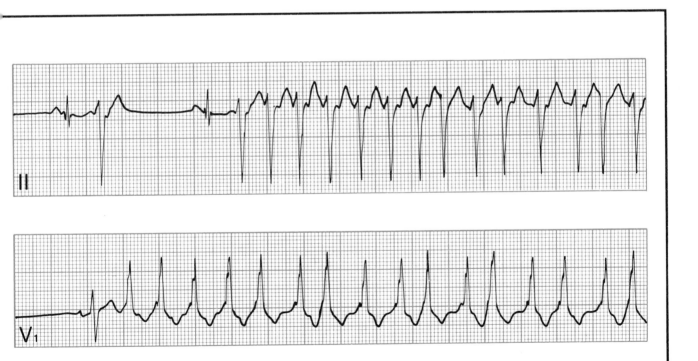

The first sinus beat is followed by a ventricular extrasystole.

The next beat is sinus and thereafter there is a rapid tachycardia. The QRS complexes are of the same configuration as the ventricular extrasystole and this is a run of ventricular tachycardia.

Lead V_1 shows the same situation—one normal sinus beat followed by a burst of ventricular tachycardia.

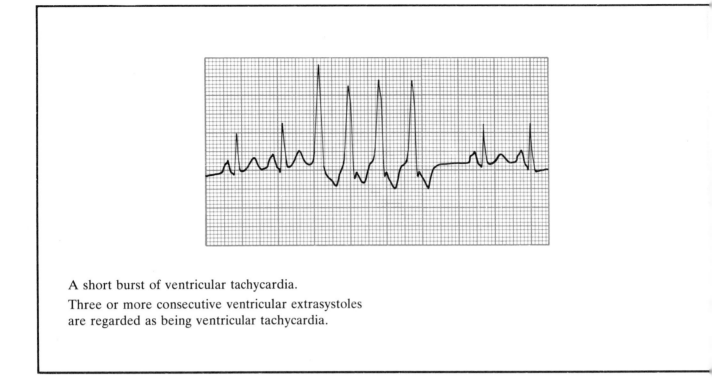

A short burst of ventricular tachycardia.

Three or more consecutive ventricular extrasystoles are regarded as being ventricular tachycardia.

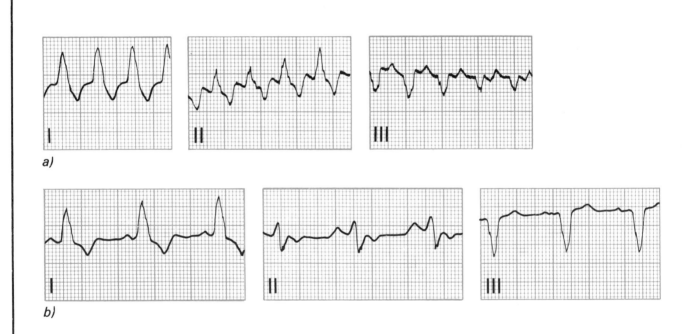

In (a) the ventricular rate is rapid, about 150 beats per minute.

The QRS complexes are broad and of abnormal shape and the possibility of ventricular tachycardia arises.

Study of the electrocardiogram (b) recorded one day later reveals that this patient has a bundle branch block when he is in sinus rhythm.

The diagnosis of the rhythm in the first tracing is therefore supraventricular tachycardia, the QRS complexes being broad because there is a bundle branch block.

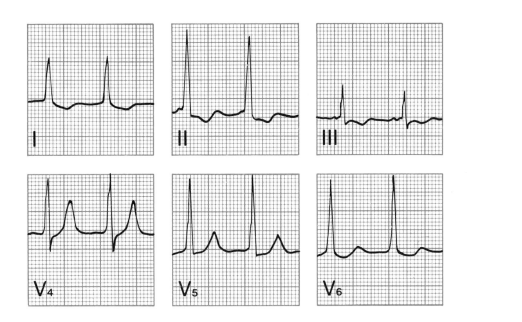

The PR interval is very short, 0.06 seconds approximately (best seen in lead II).

The QRS complexes are abnormally broad and at the beginning of the QRS there is a slurred upstroke, a delta wave (best seen in leads II, V₅ and V₆).

This is the Wolff–Parkinson–White syndrome and this patient had a normal heart.

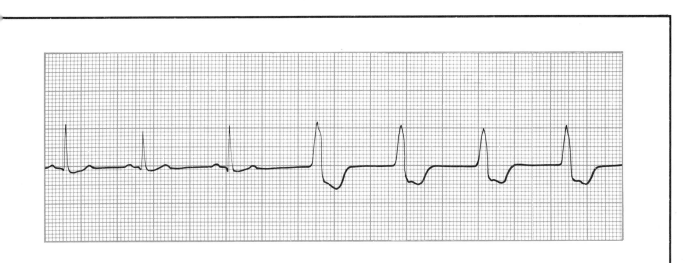

Recording taken during the first day after myocardial infarction.

After the first three sinus beats an idioventricular focus takes over the pacemaker function of the heart at a rate of about 65 beats per minute.

This is an example of idioventricular tachycardia and does not usually require antiarrhythmic drugs.

15. The Electrocardiogram in Diseases not Primarily Affecting the Heart

Endocrine Disorders

Myxoedema

From time to time the electrocardiogram provides the clue to the diagnosis, for there may be obvious electrocardiographic abnormalities in a patient who does not appear clinically to be myxoedematous.

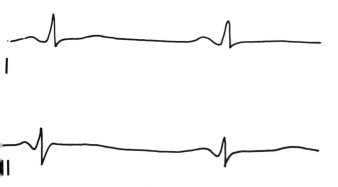

Figure 15.1.

In myxoedema, the abnormalities found on the electrocardiogram (Figure 15.1) include:

. Sinus bradycardia.

. Low amplitude T waves in all leads.

. Low amplitude QRS complexes in all leads.

Bradycardia and low amplitude T waves are usual in any patient with myxoedema, but true low voltage QRS complexes as defined later in this section are less common. Within a few weeks of the commencement of thyroid medication the electrocardiogram returns to normal.

Thyrotoxicosis

Atrial fibrillation is common in thyrotoxicosis and, when present, will be apparent on the electrocardiogram. Otherwise, the electrocardiogram is of little value in the diagnosis.

The abnormalities described in thyrotoxicosis are sinus tachycardia with tall T waves. These findings are entirely non-specific and are found in a variety of conditions, not all of which are of clinical significance.

Hypoparathyroidism

In hypoparathyroidism the low serum calcium produces a prolonged QT interval (Figure 15.2), the ST segment remaining isoelectric.

This effect is a result of the low serum calcium and the electrocardiogram becomes normal when the serum calcium level is restored to normal.

Since hypoparathyroidism may be difficult to diagnose, the electrocardiogram may provide an important clue.

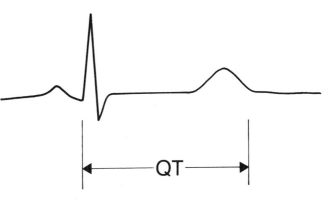

Figure 15.2.

Electrolyte Disturbances

High Serum Potassium

The electrocardiogram provides a useful indicator of the serum potassium level.

The first changes are in the T waves, and with the serum potassium in the region of 6 to 7 mEq/l(mmol/l) the T waves in the precordial leads become very tall, slender and peaked (Figure 15.3).

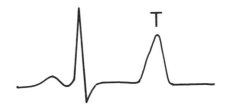

Figure 15.3. *Tall peaked T waves when the serum potassium is about 7 mEq/l(mmol/l).*

121

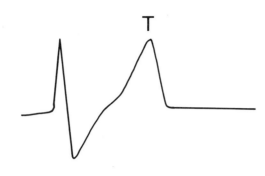

Figure 15.4. *Nodal rhythm with broad QRS complexes and tall T waves.*

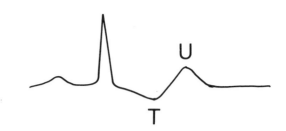

Figure 15.6. *Hypokalaemia (serum potassium around 2.5 mEq/l(mmol/l). PR interval lengthened above 0.2 seconds. ST segment depressed. T wave is now inverted. U wave is prominent but the true QT interval is normal.*

With further elevation of the serum potassium, atrial activity ceases and nodal rhythm appears (Figure 15.4).

The QRS complexes become broad, slurred and prolonged considerably above 0.12 seconds. The T waves remain tall and slender.

The serum potassium level is around 8.5 mEq/l(mmol/l).

Should the serum potassium rise still further, ventricular fibrillation or ventricular asystole will result.

Low Serum Potassium

The features of a low serum potassium are:

1. Low amplitude T waves.
2. Prominence of the U wave.

It used to be thought that low serum potassium levels produced a long QT interval but it is now known that in most cases the QT interval remains unaffected.

The appearance of a prominent U wave superimposed on the T wave produces the illusion of a prolonged QT interval (Figures 15.5 and 15.6).

The electrocardiographic appearances depend not only on the absolute level of the serum potassium but also upon the levels of the other electrolytes, particularly calcium.

The serum levels quoted corresponding to the various stages of abnormality on the electrocardiogram (Figures 15.5 and 15.6) are therefore approximations only.

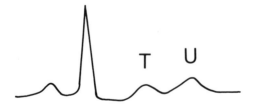

Figure 15.5. *Hypokalaemia (serum potassium below 3.5. mEq/l(mmol/l). Normal PR interval (less than 0.2 seconds). Normal duration of QRS (less than 0.09 seconds). ST segment depressed. Prominent U wave immediately following the T wave.*

High Serum Calcium Levels

The electrocardiogram is of little value in this condition Hypercalcaemia tends to shorten the QT interval, as doe digitalis medication.

Low Serum Calcium Levels

The QT interval is prolonged, sometimes markedly. Th electrocardiogram is occasionally helpful in the diagnosis as in hypoparathyroidism.

Psychological Disturbances

The electrocardiogram of a patient suffering from a anxiety state may show inversion of the T waves or slight S segment depression.

Hyperventilation, associated with anxiety and fear is prob ably partly responsible for these changes.

Once again it is emphasized that ST and T variations ar non-specific and indeed can be present in a normal heart

Intracerebral Haemorrhage

The electrocardiogram in a patient with a severe intracerebral haemorrhage may show gross T wave abnor malities.

Particularly common in subarachnoid haemorrhage, the widespread T inversion mimics myocardial infarction, ye at postmortem the heart appears completely normal.

Fortunately, from the diagnostic point of view, pathologica Q waves practically never appear.

Hypothermia

At temperatures of 30 °C bradycardia and prolongation o the QT interval are seen.

When the body temperature falls below 30 °C heart block arrhythmias and ventricular fibrillation all appear.

An extra notch on the downstroke of the R wave giving ris to an extra wave is particularly characteristic of hypother mia.

Dystrophia Myotonica and Other Muscular Dystrophies

The electrocardiogram shows some abnormality in approximately 90 per cent of all cases of dystrophia myotonica.

These include prolongation of the PR interval, atrial and ventricular arrhythmias and bundle branch block.

In most other muscular dystrophies there is a high incidence of non-specific electrocardiographic abnormality.

Abnormally Low QRS Voltages

Low voltage of the QRS complex is present when the main deflection of the QRS in any one direction from the base line is less than 5 mm in each of the standard limb leads.

Causes of low voltage include myxoedema, pericardial effusion, constrictive pericarditis and severe ischaemic heart disease.

However, low voltages in the standard leads with normal voltages in the precordial leads are not uncommon in the normal heart.

Electrical Alternans (Figure 15.7)

This finding is of no significance when it is seen during a paroxysm of tachycardia, but in other circumstances it indicates organic heart disease or pericardial effusion.

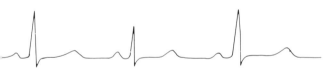

Figure 15.7. *The height of the R wave alternates every other beat.*

Summary

Myxoedema:

Associated with the following abnormalities which all revert to normal when the myxoedema is adequately treated:

1. Sinus bradycardia.
2. Low amplitude T waves.

3. Low voltage QRS complexes.

Thyrotoxicosis:

May show atrial fibrillation or sinus tachycardia with tall T waves, but the electrocardiogram is of little help in this condition.

High serum potassium:

1. Tall slender peaked T waves.
2. Nodal rhythm with prolonged QRS complexes as the potassium level continues to rise.
3. Ventricular fibrillation or ventricular asystole.

Low serum potassium:

1. Low amplitude T waves.
2. ST segment depression.
3. Prominent U waves.

High serum calcium level:

Characteristically shows a short QT interval.

Low serum calcium level:

Can occasionally be diagnosed if the electrocardiogram shows very prolonged QT intervals.

Psychological disturbances and intracerebral haemorrhage:

May show marked abnormality of the ST and T waves in the absence of organic heart disease.

Hypothermia:

Produces sinus bradycardia with a prolonged QT interval and an added wave in the QRS complex.

The muscular dystrophies:

A non-specific abnormality is common in most of the muscular dystrophies.

Low voltage QRS:

1. Present when the tallest wave in any of the limb leads is less than 5 mm.
2. Found occasionally in the normal heart.
3. Occurs in myxoedema, pericardial effusion, constrictive pericarditis and severe ischaemic heart disease.

Electrical alternans:

1. Every alternate R wave is of small amplitude.
2. In the absence of paroxysmal tachycardia electrical alternans indicates heart disease.

15. Electrocardiograms for Interpretation

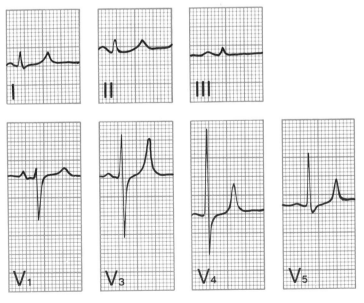

This electrocardiogram shows sinus rhythm with a normal PR interval, normal QRS complexes and a normal ST segment.

The T waves are tall, slender and peaked suggesting a high serum potassium.

The serum potassium in this patient with renal disease was 7.5 mEq/l(mmol/l).

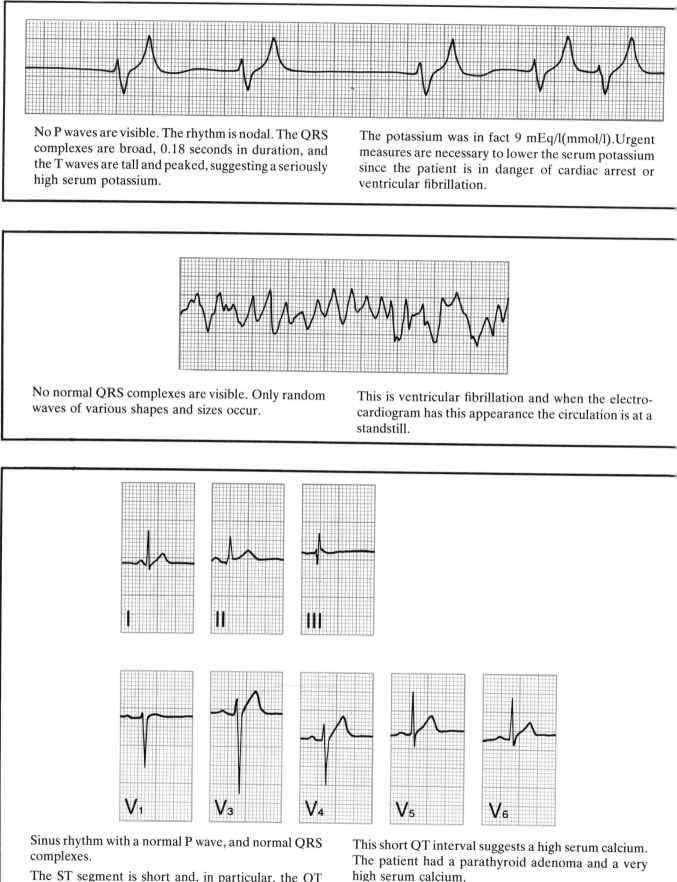

No P waves are visible. The rhythm is nodal. The QRS complexes are broad, 0.18 seconds in duration, and the T waves are tall and peaked, suggesting a seriously high serum potassium.

The potassium was in fact 9 mEq/l(mmol/l). Urgent measures are necessary to lower the serum potassium since the patient is in danger of cardiac arrest or ventricular fibrillation.

No normal QRS complexes are visible. Only random waves of various shapes and sizes occur.

This is ventricular fibrillation and when the electrocardiogram has this appearance the circulation is at a standstill.

Sinus rhythm with a normal P wave, and normal QRS complexes.

The ST segment is short and, in particular, the QT interval is abnormally short.

This short QT interval suggests a high serum calcium. The patient had a parathyroid adenoma and a very high serum calcium.

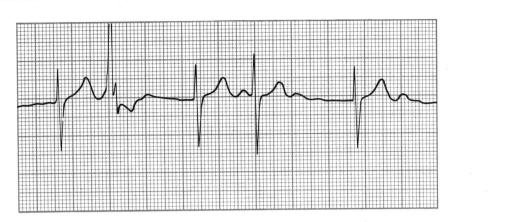

The basic rhythm here is atrial fibrillation.

The second QRS complex is a ventricular extrasystole. The wave preceding the fourth QRS complex, which at first glance seems to be a P wave, is in fact a prominent U wave. This may be confirmed by noting the prominent U waves following the last two ventricular complexes.

This electrocardiogram might suggest a low serum potassium because of the prominent U wave and the extrasystole.

The serum potassium was low, 2.8 mEq/l(mmol/l) in this patient who suffered from chronic rheumatic mitral valve disease, and this was the cause of the atrial fibrillation.

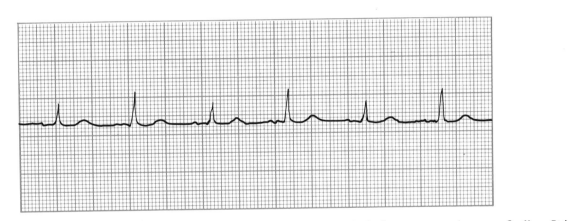

This electrocardiogram was recorded from a patient in severe left ventricular failure.

The QRS complexes are alternately large and small.

This is electrical alternans, a rather rare finding. It is more commonly associated with pericardial effusion but does occur occasionally in left ventricular failure. There was no pericardial effusion in this patient.

16. Conclusion

In this final section a scheme will be presented that should enable the practitioner to undertake the analysis of any electrocardiogram in a logical manner.

It is hoped that in addition to presenting a systematic approach this section will summarize and recall much that has been considered previously in more detail.

The study of any electrocardiogram should be carried out in a routine step-by-step process otherwise important abnormalities will be missed.

1. Heart Rate and Rhythm

The heart rate is determined by measuring the distance between the peaks of two successive R waves.

Divide the number of large squares between two successive R waves into 300 and the answer is the heart rate in beats per minute.

A ventricular rate on the resting electrocardiogram of more than 160 beats per minute or less than 50 beats per minute is unlikely to be normal sinus rhythm.

If the distance between successive R waves is always equal then the rhythm is regular. Otherwise the rhythm is irregular and a cause must be looked for.

Having determined the ventricular rate and rhythm we should next turn our attention to the P waves.

2. The P waves

The normal P wave (Figure 16.1a) is upright in leads I and II, it is less than 2.5 mm in height and about 0.08 seconds in duration (represented by two small squares on the electrocardiograph paper).

When the P wave is broad (0.12 seconds or more) and notched this indicates left atrial enlargement (Figure 16.1b)

A P wave of normal duration but tall and triangular in shape indicates right atrial hypertrophy (Figure 16.1c).

Inverted P waves in leads II and III suggest nodal rhythm (Figure 16.2).

If the P wave is inverted in lead I this usually means that the left and right arm leads have been applied incorrectly.

When these leads have not been transposed, an inverted P wave in lead I strongly suggests mirror image dextrocardia (Figure 16.3).

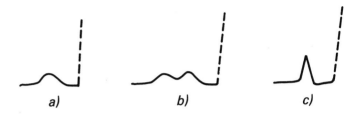

Figure 16.1. *a) Normal P wave.*

b) P mitrale indicating left atrial enlargement. Causes include: mitral valve disease and left ventricular failure.

c) P pulmonale indicating right atrial hypertrophy. Causes include: lung disease with pulmonary hypertension, pulmonary stenosis and tricuspid stenosis.

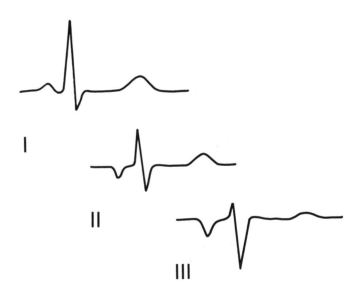

Figure 16.2. *Nodal rhythm. P waves inverted in leads II and III and the PR interval is short.*

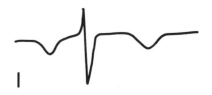

Figure 16.3. *Inverted P wave in lead 1 indicating mirror image dextrocardia.*

When the shape of the P wave has been analysed we proceed to the PR interval.

3. The PR Interval

This interval gives information on the cardiac rhythm and should always be measured from the beginning of the P wave to the beginning of the QRS complex.

The normal PR interval is not longer than 0.22 seconds and not less than 0.12 seconds.

Normal sinus rhythm is present when the P wave is upright in leads I and II, and the PR interval is constant and of normal duration (Figure 16.4).

In Figure 16.5 the P wave is of normal configuration and every P wave is followed by a QRS complex. However, the PR interval is prolonged indicating first degree heart block.

A prolonged PR interval is seen in conditions such as myocardial infarction, rheumatic fever and other forms of myocarditis and when the dosage of digitalis is excessive.

There are no P waves in Figure 16.6, but fine rapid 'f' waves are seen.

This is atrial fibrillation.

Next attention is turned to the QRS complex.

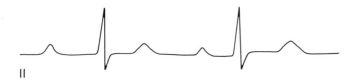

Figure 16.4.

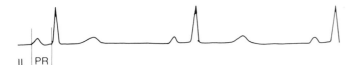

Figure 16.5.

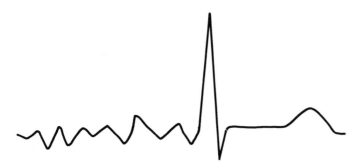

Figure 16.6.

4. The QRS Complex

The main features to be studied are the duration, amplitude and the presence or absence of pathological Q waves.

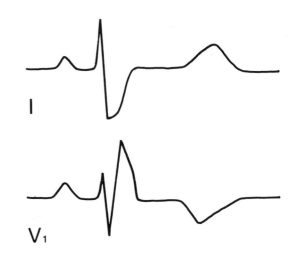

Figure 16.7. *The QRS complex is prolonged with a terminal S wave in lead I and a terminal R¹ wave in lead V₁. This is right bundle branch block.*

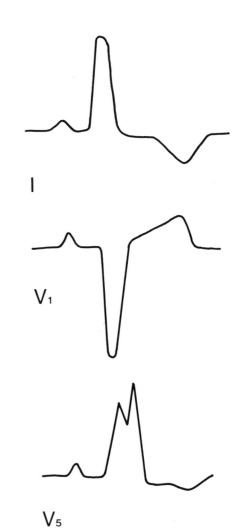

Figure 16.8. *Prolongation of the QRS complex with an absence of Q waves in leads I and V₁, and an M-shaped complex in lead V₅ indicate left bundle branch block.*

130

Duration

The normal QRS complex is less than 0.12 seconds in duration. Prolongation beyond 0.12 seconds (three small squares) indicates bundle branch block (Figures 16.7 and 16.8).

Size of the QRS Complexes

Abnormally tall R waves in V_5 with deep S waves in V_1 suggest left ventricular hypertrophy (Figure 16.9).

An R wave in lead V_1 of greater amplitude than the S wave in that lead indicates right ventricular hypertrophy (Figure 16.10).

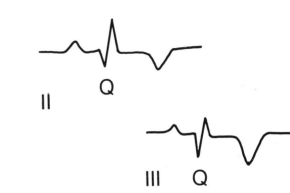

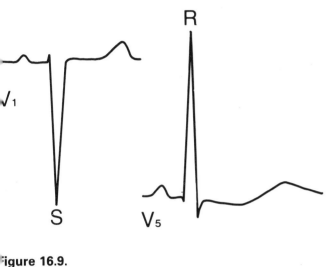

Figure 16.9.

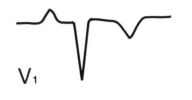

Figure 16.11. *Pathological Q waves in leads II and III indicating an inferior myocardial infarct.*

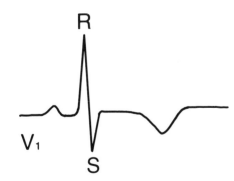

Figure 16.10. *Ratio R/S greater than 1 in lead V_1 indicating right ventricular hypertrophy.*

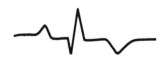

Figure 16.12. *Pathological Q waves in leads V_1, V_2 and V_3 indicating an anterior infarct.*

Presence of Pathological Q waves

Deep broad Q waves are normal in lead aVr and occasionally may be normal in leads III and V_1.

Otherwise a Q wave greater than 0.04 seconds in duration (one small square on the electrocardiogram) is almost certainly pathological (Figures 16.11 and 16.12).

5. The ST Segment

The normal ST segment is isoelectric or at most does not deviate more than 0.5 mm from the isoelectric line.

Depression of the ST segment is found in myocardial ischaemia, left ventricular hypertrophy and with digitalis treatment (Figures 16.13 and 16.14).

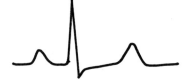

Figure 16.13. *a) Normal ST.*

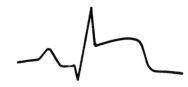

b) Acute myocardial infarct.

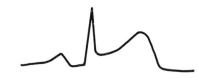

c) Acute pericarditis.

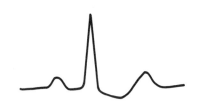

Figure 16.14. *a) Myocardial ischaemia. Flat depression of ST.*

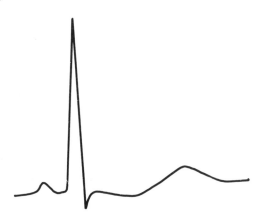

b) Digitalis effect.

c) Left ventricular hypertrophy.

6. The T wave

The T waves are affected by a large number of conditions and the changes are not specific for any disease.

T inversion occurs in myocardial infarction, left ventricular hypertrophy, chronic pericarditis, intracerebral haemorrhage, etc.

Tall peaked T waves may be normal but are also seen in myocardial ischaemia, when there is a high serum potassium level and in left ventricular enlargement.

Low voltage T waves throughout suggest myxoedema or myocardial ischaemia.

The small wave following the T wave is the U wave and is not usually of clinical significance.

Very prominent U waves suggest the possibility of a low serum potassium.

Measurement of the QT interval is occasionally helpful.

A prolonged QT interval may be found in acute carditis, low serum calcium or as a result of quinidine administration.

A shortened QT interval suggests hypercalcaemia or digitalis effect.

It is important to know if the patient is taking digitalis before attempting to draw any conclusions from abnormalities of the ST segment.

The best use of the electrocardiogram as an aid to diagnosis is made when interpretation is carried out by the physician who knows the history and findings on clinical examination in his patient.

Index